Therapeutic Intervention with Poor, Unorganized Families

From Distress to Hope

HAWORTH Marriage and the Family
Terry S. Trepper, PhD
Editor in Chief

Marriage and Family Therapy: A Sociocognitive Approach by Nathan Hurvitz and Roger A. Straus

Culture and Family: Problems and Therapy by Wen-Shing Tseng and Jing Hsu

Adolescents and Their Families: An Introduction to Assessment and Intervention by Mark Worden

Parents Whose Parents Were Divorced by R. Thomas Berner

The Effect of Children on Parents by Anne-Marie Ambert

Multigenerational Family Therapy by David S. Freeman

Therapy with Treatment Resistant Families: A Consultation-Crisis Intervention Model by William George McCown, Judith Johnson, and Associates

Developing Healthy Stepfamilies: Twenty Families Tell Their Stories by Patricia Kelley

Propagations: Thirty Years of Influence from the Mental Research Institute edited by John H. Weakland and Wendel A. Ray

Structured Exercises for Promoting Family and Group Strengths: A Handbook for Group Leaders, Trainers, Educators, Counselors, and Therapists edited by Ron McManus and Glen Jennings

Making Families Work and What to Do When They Don't: Thirty Guides for Imperfect Parents of Imperfect Children by Bill Borcherdt

Family Therapy of Neurobehavioral Disorders: Integrating Neuropsychology and Family Therapy by Judith Johnson and William McCown

Parents, Children, and Adolescents: Interactive Relationships and Development in Context by Anne-Marie Ambert

Women Survivors of Childhood Sexual Abuse: Healing Through Group Work: Beyond Survival by Judy Chew

Tales from Family Therapy: Life-Changing Clinical Experiences edited by Frank N. Thomas and Thorana S. Nelson

The Therapist's Notebook: Homework, Handouts, and Activities for Use in Psychotherapy edited by Lorna L. Hecker and Sharon A. Deacon

The Web of Poverty: Psychosocial Perspectives by Anne-Marie Ambert

Stepfamilies: A Multi-Dimensional Perspective by Roni Berger

Clinical Applications of Bowen Family Systems Theory by Peter Titelman

Treating Children in Out-of-Home Placements by Marvin Rosen

Your Family, Inc.: Practical Tips for Building a Healthy Family Business by Ellen Frankenberg

Therapeutic Intervention with Poor, Unorganized Families: From Distress to Hope by Shlomo A. Sharlin and Michal Shamai

The Residential Youth Care Worker in Action: A Collaborative, Competency-Based Approach by Robert Bertolino and Kevin Thompson

Therapeutic Intervention with Poor, Unorganized Families
From Distress to Hope

Shlomo A. Sharlin
Michal Shamai

Routledge
Taylor & Francis Group
NEW YORK AND LONDON

First Published by

The Haworth Clinical Practice Press, an imprint of The Haworth Press, Inc., 10 Alice Street, Binghamton, NY 13904-1580

Transferred to Digital Printing 2010 by Routledge
711 Third Avenue, New York NY 10017
2 Park Square, Milton Park, Abingdon, Oxon, OX14 4RN

Cover design by Jennifer M. Gaska.

The Library of Congress has cataloged the hardcover edition of this book as:

Sharlin, Sh.
Therapeutic intervention with poor, unorganized families : from distress to hope / Shlomo A. Sharlin, Michal Shamai.
p. cm.
Includes bibliographical references and index.
ISBN 0-7890-0282-5
1. Family social work. 2. Social work with the socially handicapped. 3. Problem families—Services for. 4. Poor—Services for. I. Shamai, Michal, 1949- . II. Title.
HV697.S43 1999
362.82—dc21 99-34432
CIP

ISBN: 0-7890-0283-3 (pbk.)

Publisher's Note
The publisher has gone to great lengths to ensure the quality of this reprint but points out that some imperfections in the original may be apparent.

CONTENTS

PART IV: INTERVENTION TECHNIQUES

ABOUT THE AUTHORS

Shlomo A. Sharlin, PhD, is Professor and Director at The Center for Research and Study of the Family, and former Dean of the School of Social Work at the University of Haifa, Israel. Dr. Sharlin has extensive experience in youth and family psychotherapy and has published numerous articles in scholarly international journals. He has lectured and counseled on youth and the family in many countries, including the United States. In 1986, Dr. Sharlin was appointed Director of the Center for Research and Study of the Family at the University of Haifa. During the past decade, he has directed numerous projects with families and youth in distress, has developed techniques for intervention with unorganized and disadvantaged families, and has developed adolescent suicide prevention programs. Recently, Dr. Sharlin conducted a major study for the State of Israel on family policy. In addition, Dr. Sharlin is a board member of the International Family Therapy Association.

Michal Shamai, PhD, is Director of the Social Work Department at Tel-Chai College in Israel. She is also a clinical lecturer at the School of Social Work at the University of Haifa. Dr. Shamai worked and supervised at the Kibbutz Child and Family Clinic and for several years she was the Director of the Regional Center for Family Therapy Training and Intervention in Haifa. There she developed the first Israeli clinic specializing in the treatment of domestic violence. During the past decade, she has directed and collaborated on research and clinical projects relating to families in extreme distress, domestic violence, and families living in a state of uncertainty as a result of the peace process. Dr. Shamai has had her articles on these issues published in several scholarly international journals.

Senior Editor's Comments

Almost all therapists at one time or another, no matter what their discipline or orientation, work with poor families. Usually, we see poorer families during our graduate training, since most of our practicum and internship experiences occur in university-, community agency-, or state-run mental health facilities that have primarily poor families as their clients. It has been noted by many that poor families, with their increased vulnerabilities to behavioral and mental health problems, should probably be treated by those clinicians and social workers with the *most* experience, not those with the least, such as practicum students and clinical interns. However, no matter who provides the treatment, one problem has been the dearth of training material specifically focused on interventions with poor families.

This magnificent book, by two international experts on family therapy interventions with poor families, is one of the first to offer a comprehensive analysis, assessment, and intervention program for those who work with this population. Sharlin and Shamai have done extensive research on interventions with poor families, and from their studies, they have developed a model that is not only empirically supported but clinically relevant. Therapists are rarely offered such a complete and scientifically sound program of intervention in any specialty area, much less one that focuses on working with this ubiquitous and challenging population.

Therapeutic Intervention with Poor, Unorganized Families: From Distress to Hope is unique in that it can be used in a variety of professional contexts. The book is a fascinating and complete sociology text on the structures of poor families, as well as an overview and guide for workers in social service agencies to better understand the complexities of poor families. The book can also be used as a complete treatment manual in mental health agencies that provide clinical services to poor families. Finally, the book will be of great interest to sociology, psychology, and social work researchers who are studying functional and dysfunctional structures of vulnerable families.

Whichever group you are in, I know you will find *Therapeutic Intervention with Poor, Unorganized Families* to be useful. It is well-written, tightly organized, and quite intriguing. Whether you are currently working with poor families or will be in the future, this book will be an essential part of your professional library.

Terry S. Trepper, PhD
Editor in Chief
The Haworth Clinical Practice Press

Foreword

Poor, disorganized, "multiproblem" families have always been at the core of social work's attention. Friendly visitors, the nineteenth-century predecessors of professional social workers, attempted by precept and example to uplift such families from their dire straits. Occasionally they succeeded, but most often they failed. In the century of programs that followed, we have tried numerous approaches with this challenging clientele. As knowledge has accumulated and new methods have been introduced, our success rate has perhaps improved. However, all that has been accomplished is still dwarfed by the enormity of the problems these families present.

In this book, Shlomo Sharlin and Michal Shamai bring us up to date on the approaches taken with this population and offer promising directions for further efforts. After a scholarly review of past attempts to serve multiproblem families, they describe an approach they have developed and used in Israel to serve such families, whom they aptly call "families in extreme distress." Readers in the United States will immediately recognize such families and can readily apply the authors' ideas and methods to their own locales.

Indeed, they will find much to apply. With a forthright and engaging style, Sharlin and Shamai present a well-seasoned, practical model for work with families in extreme distress. Drawing on developments in structural family, solution-focused, and narrative therapies, as well as on more traditional methods, they craft a well-structured, eclectic approach directed at building on families' strengths. The model itself represents a major step forward in efforts to help such families. In addition, it presents a number of specific advances that merit comment.

Perhaps the most intriguing of the authors' contributions is their notion that practitioners can inadvertently take on the characteristics of the families they seek to help. Thus, a family's disorganization, lack of boundaries, low frustration tolerance, hopelessness, and aggression can engender similar reactions in social workers. As a result, both the family and its helpers can be caught in a downward spiral—a "coalition of despair." The authors provide an engrossing account of how these coalitions are formed and how they can be overcome. Special preparation of practitioners, use of teams, and skilled supervision are among their remedies.

The assessment of multiproblem families is a complex task, given the many facets of their functioning that need to be taken into account. Another contribution of the volume is a relatively simple scale that practitioners can complete from data they should ordinarily obtain from early interviews with the family. The Family in Extreme Distress Scale, which the authors developed through a number of studies, provides the practitioner with a systematic profile of the family's functioning across nine areas. The scale can not only facilitate clinical work but also provide an evaluation of changes associated with service.

Traditionally, it has been assumed that most multiproblem families "need" long-term services because of their severe dysfunctions. Yet, we know that most such families have been unwilling to accept lengthy courses of treatment. Some end service "prematurely," once their immediate crisis has been resolved; others reject from the outset any sustained helping effort. Moreover, in long-term treatment, there is the risk that all participants will be consumed in an interminable relationship that attempts to deal with everything and accomplishes nothing. One solution seems to be structured, well-focused, time-limited service that offers intensive help with a family's most pressing issues, while teaching communication, parenting, and problem-solving skills that will enable the family to cope independently with the inevitable difficulties of the future. However, many such families may need more than is provided by rigidly limited short-term programs. Sharlin and Shamai offer a reasonable compromise: a three-month period of intensive service, followed by a three-month maintenance period, and then another three months of intensive service, if necessary. This kind of program structure is in line with much contemporary thinking about the best way of serving many types of clients faced with chronic problems of living: the use of brief service episodes on an as-needed basis, interspersed with periods of monitoring.

A dominant characteristic of contemporary social work practice is its eclecticism. In my view, this development is inevitable, as we begin to shed our allegiances to the hundreds of different schools that populate the treatment landscape. More and more practitioners have come to recognize that loyalty to a particular approach excessively limits the kinds of interventions that might be profitably used in any particular case at hand. However, eclectic practice may lack the kind of coherence needed to achieve optimal results. One solution has been the development of integrative practice models that organize diverse practice methods within particular theoretical frameworks. Sharlin and Shamai offer a different solution—the concept of a "toolbox" of practice methods. In developing their own eclectic approach, they have selected methods that appear to work for them in their interventions with families in extreme distress. They deliberately eschew complex, integrative formulations at a theoretical level. Their main organizing principle is "If it works, then use it!" What they have achieved is a practical, but thoughtful, eclecticism fashioned by the criterion of perceived effectiveness. Their toolbox is expandable, depending on what else is found to work. The tools can be sorted out and classified after they have been selected, and a theoretical rationale for their selection can then be built, as the authors do quite well. This simple bottom-up approach to model construction challenges conventional thinking about integration in which emphasis is placed on complex top-down theorizing. If the bottom-up approach is used to develop a model for a particular population, then a focus on the population itself can facilitate the creation of a coherent rationale for the methods selected. The authors' model offers a case in point.

Most programs designed to serve families in extreme distress are never rigorously evaluated. Of those which have been, many have failed to demonstrate positive effects. It is indeed the exception for a model to be presented with sound empirical credentials, that is, with evidence of positive effects derived from a controlled test. The present model clearly is such an exception. A rigorous, randomized design was used to determine if families treated by the authors' approach would have better outcomes than a group of control families. The experimental families did in fact surpass the controls on several key measures. The study illustrates not only the importance of providing empirical backing for one's innovation, but also the process that is likely to produce such evidence. In particular, the authors made use of a developmental research process in which informal trials, including a substantial pilot test, were used to improve their interventions prior to the controlled experiment. They offer a rare, but gratifying, example of how to build and test innovative service programs.

Sharlin and Shamai have presented a state-of-the-art approach to working with families in extreme distress. In so doing, they have contributed a fascinating conceptualization of practitioner-client interaction, new methods of assessment, a simple, but ingenious, method of constructing an eclectic practice model, and an exemplar of intervention research. Read on!

William J. Reid
Distinguished Professor
State University of New York at Albany

Preface

The writing of this book, the project described in it, and the dream that gave birth to the project were shared by the authors, who collaborated and contributed equally to every aspect and nuance of the research and execution.

Both of us are social workers and family therapists with a firm belief in society's responsibility toward its members. We believe that the historical social work commitment toward the poor has remained valid and that the different views in family therapy approaches are relevant to intervention with the poor. We recognize, with a great deal of respect, poor families' struggle for survival and their desire to provide their children with better lives.

When Ester Solomon, who was, in 1990, director of the Department of Individual and Family Services of the Ministry of Labor and Social Affairs in Haifa and the northern region of Israel, suggested that "we do something with these families, whom no one has been able to help" (they were all well known to the Department of Social Services), we were very enthusiastic to accept the challenge.

Very early in our project, we realized that the professionals authorized to work with multiproblem families also shared some of the families' feelings of despair. It was obvious to us, therefore, that to help multiproblem families, we would first have to encourage and reinforce the social workers, family therapists, and other professionals involved in their commitment and ability to help the poor. It should be mentioned here that, since most interventions with the poor are carried out by social workers, the project took place at the Department of Social Services in the northern part of Israel.

In this book, we describe our learning experience with poor families as well as with the professionals involved. While the families taught us about their own lives and the way to approach and help them, we, the professionals, tried to present them with new alternatives. Social workers shared with us their skills and experiences, as well as their frustrations and feelings of despair. We, in turn, shared with them our professional knowledge regarding family intervention. We thus created a context of mutual trust between families and social workers, which led to more effective working relationships. Our academic background helped us to evaluate the process systematically and to summarize and present it to professionals at international conferences, who strongly encouraged us to share our experience with the professional community at large. These professionals had always considered working with the poor a very complex and difficult task. We accepted their challenge, which resulted in this book.

Part I of the book deals with theory and practical application, which represents the historical knowledge that is the basis for our project. In Chapter 1, we describe the development of the concepts of "poor families" and "multiproblem" families, as well as the criteria for preferring the term "families in extreme distress" (FED). Chapter 2 describes the acquired intervention experience and the various intervention approaches used with this population since the 1940s.

Part II of the book goes from theory to practice. Chapter 3 describes the phenomenon defined as a "coalition of despair" that occurs between families and the social workers or other professionals involved. It discusses also the ways to overcome this "coalition of despair" and turn it into a "coalition of hope." This represents a very important turning point for family therapists' and social workers' ability to effectively work with families in extreme distress. Based on this work, as well as our previous knowledge and experience, we developed a therapeutic model, which includes the therapeutic team, structured intervention, and home-based sessions.

Part III explains an assessment scale that has been developed to define the specific problems in each family. This scale also allows evaluation of therapy and follow-up on therapeutic outcome.

Part IV deals with intervention techniques. Chapters 5 and 6 describe the "toolbox" that consists of multiple intervention techniques. The toolbox offers a variety of alternatives for intervention; it does not limit us to one approach, but rather reinforces the concept of using every tool found to be effective. In the content analysis of the intervention process, we describe two main types of techniques. One category is "preparatory techniques," described in Chapter 5; the other is "change-oriented techniques," described in Chapter 6. We find that most of the techniques used belong to the preparatory techniques group. Chapter 7 describes a networking process in which different agencies in the community are invited to take part in a multiprofessional team. The rationale for forming such a team for the purpose of therapeutic intervention with FED is demonstrated. Chapter 8 portrays the study of one family who participated in the project, the L. family, describing the process in detail, including dialogue quoted from the meetings. The process is summarized with a subjective evaluation by the family itself and by the therapeutic team. Chapter 9 concentrates on the supervisory process involving family therapists and social workers taking part in the project, with special emphasis on issues concerning supervision of practitioners working with families in extreme distress. One such issue is the role of the supervisor as the "container" of the social worker's state of despair and sense of being overwhelmed.

Part V presents the process and research evaluation. Chapter 10 describes the reasons and goals of the project. It includes a detailed description of the pilot study upon which the structure and procedures used in the therapeutic model were designed. Chapter 11 describes quantitative and qualitative evaluations, with the primary noticeable progress found in problem-solving skills. The qualitative evaluation reports point to positive changes, such as improved functioning and renewed hope, in almost all the families in the experimental group.

Part VI of the book is the epilogue; Chapter 12 includes a summary of our project, questions about the future direction of interventions with families in extreme distress, and attempts to answer some of these questions.

We believe that we have succeeded in integrating theory, practice, and research. It is our hope that the project does not end here, but that it will be used by social workers and family therapists as a resource to encourage intervention with families in extreme distress. We also hope that it will offer a useful base of knowledge to which social workers and family therapists will add their own subjective experiences, consistent with the specific cultural backgrounds of their clients.

We hope that our efforts will have been worthwhile and that the book will prove stimulating to our readers.

Shlomo A. Sharlin
Michal Shamai

Acknowledgments

We would like to thank the many people who stayed with us during this entire project. First on the list are the families who took part in the project, who opened their hearts and homes to us, were ready to join us in this challenge, and agreed to intervention alternatives that had the potential to rekindle hope in their lives. Next, we want to extend our deep appreciation to the staff at the Department of Social Services in Tiberias and Beth-Shean, who were ready to invest time and energy, were open for the new alternatives suggested, and also shared the workers' feelings of despair. We also thank the staff of the Departments of Social Services in Hazor-Haglilit, Yokneam, and Hadera, who allowed us to reexamine some of our experiences. Many thanks and our deep appreciation go to Dvorit Gilad-Smolinsky and Pnina Blitz, family therapists, and to Hedva Rubin, project coordinator, for their creativity and dedication during the project and the evaluation process.

Above all, we would like to thank Ester Solomon and Shlomo Medina, of the Ministry of Labor and Social Affairs, who made this project possible by believing in the commitment and the responsibility of society toward all its members, as well as for believing that social work is the profession most suited to this responsibility.

We would also like to express our appreciation to our colleague and good friend Florence Kaslow, who, with her endless energy and spirit, encouraged us to publish this material and put us in touch with The Haworth Press.

Our many thanks to the staff at the Center for Research and Study of the Family for their tremendous support: to Jeannette Solomon, without whose dedication, typing, retyping, and editing, this book would not have been possible; to Sharon Woodrow for her excellent editing; to Victor Moin for helping with the artwork; and to Liora Kalish and Miri Lerner for their help throughout.

Last, but not least, we thank the members of our families for their patience and support: To the Sharlins, Nurit, Ephie, Inbal and Sela,

Ettie and Ayelet. To the Shamais, Shalom, Gal, Ye'ellah, Yonat, and Aviv. We thank you for supporting us along the way and for resigning yourselves to weekends turned into workdays. Deepest gratitude goes to Michal Shamai's late father, Yerachmiel Galster, who provided a lifelong example of dedication to others.

PART I:
INTRODUCTION TO THE PROBLEM

Chapter 1

The Distress: A Social Problem of Families in Extreme Distress and Multiproblem Families

Poverty can be found as far back as the Old Testament: ". . . but the seventh year thou shalt let it rest and lie fallow that the poor of thy people may eat" (Exodus 23:11). Used as a precursor for the modern welfare state, the term poor has remained with us ever since, never leaving society's agenda. More specifically, we should mention the Poor Laws of 1598 and 1601 and the development of Marxist ideas and ideology to combat poverty and social injustice. Through the centuries, different approaches have been used, but it was only during the second part of the twentieth century that systematic, scientific, and clinical attention was given to this issue.

On the threshold of the twenty-first century, we focus on the second half of the twentieth century in an attempt to understand, clarify, and describe what we have learned during the past fifty years. The term most used during this period to describe the poor has been multiproblem families, first used and introduced by Isaac Hoffman, research director of the Wilder Foundation in St. Paul, Minnesota. He used the term to define families with serious problems in more than one of the following areas: health, economic behavior, social adjustment, and recreational needs (Buell and associates, 1952; Geismar and La Sorte, 1964).

Hoffman's definition of multiproblem families referred more to specific family problems than to family characteristics. However, other descriptive terms have been used in the literature to designate multiproblem families, such as deprived (Pavenstedt, 1965), disorganized (Minuchin and Montalvo, 1968), hard-core (Kaplan, 1986; Schlesinger, 1970; Tomlinson and Peters, 1981), disadvantaged (Aponte, 1994; Lorion, 1978), defeated (Rosenfeld, 1989), and poor families (Tomlinson and Peters, 1981). Each definition points to a different family characteristic, shedding light on different aspects of the same family condition. Together they demonstrate the complexity of this social phenomenon. We will attempt to analyze and understand what has been learned about the phenomenon since the 1940s.

HISTORICAL REVIEW: FROM MULTIPROBLEM FAMILIES TO FAMILIES IN EXTREME DISTRESS (FED)

The 1940s Through the 1960s

After World War II, during the late 1940s, we see the first attempts at analyzing social phenomena from a scientific point of view. Empirical studies of various social problems were vigorously embarked upon, with multiproblem families among them. The basic idea of social problems can be found in Charles Booth's writings. At the beginning of the century, Charles Booth (1903) wrote about poverty in London in the 1880s and 1890s, as well as at the beginning of the twentieth century. He regarded poverty as a central problem and the cause of many others. Although poverty was considered a political issue affecting social policy, it was also associated with personal attitudes such as laziness and indolence. By the same token, society and the government, as well as the poor families themselves, were held responsible for their condition. Consequently, social planning strategies tried to solve all problems stemming from poverty by providing financial assistance.

Isaac Hoffman first introduced the term multiproblem family based on the results of an extensive study carried out in St. Paul, Minnesota, on families receiving social services in that area. The study was called "The Family Unit Report" (Buell and associates, 1952). Conclusions of the study formulated an important equation, which demonstrated that poor families with severe and multiple problems who received help from a variety of social agencies were indeed multiproblem families. Subsequently, to be identified as a multiproblem family, the family had to be considered poor and constantly assisted by various social agencies. This equation remained practically unchallenged for at least twenty years.

Many prominent social analysts of the 1950s and 1960s, such as Chilman (1966), Galbraith (1958), Harrington (1962), Miller (1962), and Lewis (1959, 1961, 1966), examined the concept of poverty from a different perspective. Lewis (1959), for instance, was the first to use the concept of a "poverty culture." He wrote:

> Poverty becomes a dynamic factor which affects participation in the larger national culture and creates a subculture of its own. . . . It seems to me that the culture of poverty cuts across regional, rural-urban and even national boundaries. For example, I am impressed with the remarkable similarities in family structure, the nature of kinship ties, the quality of husband-wife and parent-child relations, time orientation, spending patterns, value systems and the sense of community. . . ." (p. 16)

Thus, he did not emphasize the family's financial status, but rather its way of life, interorganization, and relationship with society.

Similar to Lewis, Harrington (1962) also pointed out that multiproblem families, in addition to being extremely poor, also operate with their own sets of values and norms that are totally different from the normative way of life in society at large. Miller (1962) emphasized multiproblem families' instability and their lack of financial security. Also documented in the literature are the distinct personality characteristics created by poverty. Frankenstein (1969) and Lewis (1966) singled out weak ego, low self-esteem, lack of basic trust, and a dependent personality. Chilman (1968) described a sense of fatalism expressed by people living in severe poverty, which can lead to passivity or to the use of force and aggression.

In spite of the extensive literature about poverty accumulated during the 1950s and early 1960s, it soon appeared that not every poor family, not even the extremely poor, became a multiproblem family. It also became clear that poverty was only one condition among many others that drove a family into a multiproblem existence and that the phenomenon of the multiproblem family was not the result of economic hardship alone. A multiplicity of variables in different areas were instrumental in reaching the high level of dysfunction that maintained the extreme distress through time and generations (Gans, 1963). To distinguish between severely poor families and multiproblem families, two important attempts were made at classifying multiproblem families. The first, embarked upon by Community Research Associates, included five criteria (Spencer, 1963b): (1) failure in the functioning of the mother, (2) failure in the functioning of the father, (3) failure in the functioning of the siblings, (4) failure in marital adjustment, and (5) economic deprivation and grossly inadequate housing. The New York City Council Board studied 150 families using the previous classification and concluded that 87 percent of multiproblem families studied failed in at least three categories and 35 percent failed in all five, but the study did not specify which three categories. The second attempt was made by the State Charities Aid Association of New York, which put forward the following classification (Spencer, 1963b): (1) multiplicity of problems, (2) chronicity of need, (3) resistance to treatment, and (4) handicapping attitudes, such as alienation from the community, hostility, and suspicion of authority.

Reissman, Cohen, and Pearl (1964) argued that multiproblem families, in addition to being poor, could not or would not adopt middle-class norms and values and rejected any association with professional unions. Contrary to Lewis (1959), Pavenstedt (1965) stated that, although multiproblem families have many psychological and social problems, as well as high levels of disorganization and pathology, multiple-problem families "do not belong to a 'culture,' having neither traditions nor institutions, ethnic ties or active religious affiliations to hold them together. In fact, we speak of Multiproblem Families as a group only because of common family life patterns and a kind of peripheral social existence" (p. 10).

An important publication and a step forward in social research is Schlesinger's book *The Multi-Problem Family* (1963). This book contains a review of annotated bibliographies from different countries around the world, spanning the late 1940s until the early 1960s. In the first chapter, Spencer (1963b) points out the vagueness of the multiproblem family concept, its tremendous scope, and the difficulty in defining it. It is, therefore, almost impossible to include all the different facets of this social phenomenon in a single, clear, and precise definition. Spencer claims that "The multiproblem family is easier to describe than to define, and the majority of definitions found in literature are in fact descriptions of characteristics derived mainly from observation and experience in the field of social work. . . . Our knowledge of causation still remains vague and imprecise" (p. 7). Spencer provides a long list of typical multiproblem family characteristics, such as large family size, the high rate of mobility, isolation, alienation, destructive parent-child relationships, and chronic dependence on community services combined with an aversion for help, delinquency, disorganization, instability, and emotional immaturity. Yet, we do not find all of these problems in one family. Different families suffer from different symptoms. The exact combination of problems that creates a multiproblem family is still unclear.

Multiproblem families are recognizable mostly in countries with high living standards, since ". . . Western society's high standards of wealth and expectations of social welfare services has brought to public attention a difficult social problem that had previously remained concealed" (Spencer, 1963b, p. 3). In a survey of 400,000 families in Great Britain, for example, Scott (1956) found that more than 3,000 families suffered from low intelligence, mental illness, criminal behavior, drinking and gambling, cruelty toward children, repeated hospitalization, persistent quarreling and truancy, overcrowded and intolerable living conditions, and failure to respond to help offered by different social services.

In summary, it was during the 1940s, 1950s, and 1960s that the first attempts were made to analyze, define, and classify the phenomenon of multiproblem families, with an extensive list of characteristics being attributed to such families. However, some questions should be raised in this regard: How long is that list, and which criteria are relevant? Are any of the factors preconditions? From these descriptions, the existence of severe impairment in the functioning of the family and the inability of its members to cope is quite obvious. It is also apparent that multiproblem families suffer from a multiplicity of problems, such as poor relationships among family members, as well as with the immediate community. Most of the literature of the 1960s and 1970s that attempts to address these questions describes projects concerning various poverty issues, especially in the field of social work. It was mainly social workers, employed in diverse social services, who provided descriptions of real-life experiences with their multiproblem clients.

The 1970s

During the 1970s, social scientists started to break down the different categories and descriptions that had been previously coined to define or classify multiproblem families; they then proceeded to elaborate and further explore each of the categories. During this period, new definitions to describe multiproblem families appeared in the literature. We find the terms disorganized, which is used to describe a high level of disorganization (Frairberg, 1978), unmotivated (Frairberg, 1978), self-defeating (Schlesinger, 1970); and hopeless (Frairberg, 1978), describing an atmosphere of apathy and withdrawal. The phrase "hard to reach" refers to multiproblem families' resistance to treatment (Frairberg 1978; Schlesinger, 1970; Spencer, 1963b). Finally, since they are always on the lowest rung of society, they are also defined as disadvantaged (Lorion, 1978). These new labels, in contrast to the term multiproblem family, tend to describe the families' emotional state.

The perspective of these definitions has since changed from mere description to include causality. Furthermore, since we know that different problems in multiproblem families impact on one another, we cannot suggest a linear cause-and-effect relationship, but rather a circular connection among the various problems. Based on the literature of the 1970s, one can pose the following questions: What is the meaning of failure in the roles of parents and children? What is the significance of multiproblem families' dependence on social services, and why are they so resistant to help? The discussion on these issues will be treated more extensively in the following chapter.

Parental Role Failure and Marital Adjustment Failure

Polansky, Borgman, and DeSaix (1972), in their book *Roots of Futility,* speculate on what makes different people, or families, react in singular ways to their life experiences. Polansky asks, "Why is it that we meet a child on AFDC (Aid to Families with Dependent Children) who is skinny, barefoot, and unkempt, while half a mile away is another child, also on AFDC, but infinitely better cared for?" (p. 3). The question is highly relevant, and can be illustrated by the following two examples:

> John Ash, 17 years old, is a dropout by necessity, not by choice. His girl is pregnant. . . . He has to get married and go to work, if he can get a job. The place John calls home is an undersized apartment. . . . On television a white child tempts them with toys they will never enjoy. . . . For John's brother, Calvin, age eleven, reading is a torturously slow affair. Nathaniel's only playground is the street. Calvin's older brother, John, has one ambition: to start a youth labor union. . . . He is afraid that his ideas and all his ambitions are going to fade, but he will keep on plugging. "You try to move a little faster," he says, "so the world won't leave you behind with your head in your hands." (Leinwand, 1968, pp. 54-56)

> There were seven children in the family and her father earned $12 a week. They had a three-room, cold water flat and no lights. . . . Her parents fought constantly. Her father was ill-tempered and gave her mother a hard time. Her mother was a nice person but had to work too hard. The mother indulged in much outside sexual activity as well as probably being epileptic. . . . He (the father) tried to molest her several times. . . . She always had to work and give the wages to her father which he immediately drank up. (Geismar and La Sorte, 1964, pp. 141-142)

In the first example, we find a family struggling with severe economic problems and deprivation. However, there is ambition and, more important, hope for a better future. We see a family that, despite tremendous obstacles, attempts to challenge what appears to be its fate. In the second example, one can almost sense the despair. "We didn't have anything," says one of the family members, and by that, she refers to "the economic situation but also to a complete absence of family cohesiveness" (Geismar and La Sorte, 1964, p. 141).

As we have seen, even if both parents are present, they fail in their parental roles. Both Mazer (1972) and Chilman (1973) emphasize that in multiproblem families, many couples marry when the wife is already pregnant, and since they have little family-planning knowledge, if any at all, they end up having many children, one after the other. They also typically marry very young as an escape from their own families. In many cases, in addition to the fact that they are neither prepared nor qualified to become parents, these couples do not really want to have children. It is no surprise, therefore, that they have difficulty functioning as parents, being, themselves, children who have children. Herein lies the essence of the vicious cycle, perpetuating itself from one generation to the next (Polansky, Borgman, DeSaix, 1970; Polansky, Borgman, and DeSaix, 1972). Minuchin and associates (1967), in their book *Families of the Slums,* point out the need for parents in any family to share in the responsibilities of parenthood in a complementary manner. Such sharing does not generally exist in multiproblem families, since both parents lack the skills of competent functioning. Parental responsibilities are often transferred to the older siblings or to all the children in the family. Sometimes, very young children are forced to take on responsibilities that are well beyond their capabilities (Marans and Lourie, 1967).

In many multiproblem families, at least one member of the family is constantly looking for work. Since many of the men have either criminal records or some kind of addiction (drug, alcohol, or gambling), it is often the women who find work, bringing about a role reversal that greatly affects the relationship between the parents (Pettigrew, 1964). The men sense their failure as fathers and in their role as head of the family. The mothers, on the other hand, are overworked and overloaded with responsibilities, making them unable to invest time or energy in their children, who, as a result, are deprived of much-needed emotional support (Polansky, DeSaix, and Sharlin, 1972; Polansky et al., 1981).

It is important to note that the reversal of traditional roles described here is not equally balanced. Although many women work outside the home, it is in addition to their housekeeping responsibilities, while the husbands do not contribute to child care or housekeeping chores. Unemployed, they remain idle, easily falling prey to alcoholism, drug abuse, or other criminal activity. Since the fathers in multiproblem families typically do not provide for their families, their role as "man of the house" is greatly impaired, and in an attempt to assert their masculinity, they may become violent toward their wives or their children.

Although it is clear that parents can hardly function under such conditions, research has largely neglected the study of these fathers, focusing mainly on the mothers. The mothers are often described as apathetic, hopeless, and in extreme despair. Polansky and colleagues (1972) call it "The apathy-futility syndrome" (p. 54), citing it as a possible cause of child neglect.

> The characteristic effect of the apathy-futility syndrome is the deep sense of futility, accompanied by massive inhibition, giving rise to a far-reaching anesthesia or numbness. Behaviorally, there is a generalized slowing down and a straining towards immobility. . . . Impoverishment in relationships is accompanied by reticence, especially in speech. (Polansky, Borgman, and DeSaix, 1972, pp. 54-55)

Evidence of poor communication in multiproblem families is very common in the literature (Bernstein, 1960, 1961, 1962, 1964; Marans and Lourie, 1967; Minuchin et al., 1967; Minuchin and Montalvo, 1968). Communication, either between the spouses or between parents and children, is mostly of an informative nature and very concise. They only share very basic, unsophisticated information, hardly listening to one another and attempting to speak at the same time. The couples argue and quarrel a great deal, with potentially violent results (Minuchin et al., 1967).

Parents in multiproblem families not only fail in their parental roles and their family relationships but also in their relations with the immediate community as well. The multiple-problem family actually suffers from extensive social isolation (Schlesinger, 1970; Spencer, 1963b). Economic instability forces the family to move very frequently, thus making a supportive social network almost unattainable (Spencer, 1963a). Multiproblem family members do not spend any free time together as a family. The men socialize with other men, usually in the streets, and often engage in criminal activity as a means of making some easy money to support their addictions. The women, on the other hand, do not have much leisure time and rely on what is described in the literature as the "multiplicity of mothers" (Chilman, 1966). This means that children are being raised either by the extended family, their siblings, or their neighbors. As a result, little emotional bonding is established between the mother and her children.

Is there any chance at all for children growing up in a multiproblem family to break the vicious cycle and eventually make a success of their lives? There is little evidence of this in the literature. The family's instability and the lack of normal parental role models have a very strong impact on the children of multiproblem families. According to Marans and Lourie (1967), children show fearful obedience in the presence of their parents, but in their absence, they turn to violent behavior, such as the destruction of property or violent fights with other children. They grow up in an atmosphere of fear and instability, with no alternatives. Their home environment dictates their behavior, offering no explanations or emotional support. There is no time for play, no time for childhood. These children grow up on their own from a very early age, and there is little hope for them to develop a stable and mature personality. They suffer from neglect, low self-esteem, immaturity, and a lack of self-confidence, and they are likely to develop personality disorders later in life (Bronfenbrenner, 1968; Geismar, 1973; Marans and Lourie, 1967; Mazer, 1972; Minuchin, 1970; Minuchin et al., 1967; Polansky, DeSaix, and Sharlin, 1972). Not surprisingly, research indicates that many of these children have been physically abused (Minuchin et al., 1967; Pavestedt, 1965). In the following example, given by Polansky, Borgman, and DeSaix (1972), we can feel the atmosphere in which these children grow up:

> The first child born to the Archers died in infancy because "she just wasn't able to make it. . . ." The second child was an attractive six-year-old with beautiful blue-green eyes, dark curly hair, and a wiry little body. In her first year at school she presented two problems: first, her mother did not really want her to leave home to go to school; second, she took home everything she could get her hands on . . . even possessions of other children which appealed to her. . . . Sue Ella frequently complained of toothache and happily stayed home from school. (p. 13)

The 1980s and 1990s

During the 1980s and 1990s, the term multiproblem families is almost absent from the literature, pointing to a change in focus. Many of the studies deal with a narrow and very specific multiproblem family problem, whether it be drug abuse, delinquency, alcoholism, or child neglect. Although these are all individual consequences of a life in extreme distress, attempts to deal with multiproblem families as a whole are quite rare (Hanson and Carta, 1996; Kaplan, 1984).

Mental Health and the Multiproblem Family

The relationship between mental health and the multiproblem family has been discussed in the literature since the late 1950s. A positive correlation was found between individual mental illness and family deterioration and deprived socioeconomic conditions (Pasamanick, 1959). Beyond this claim, other studies emphasized the correlation between families who experience severe economic deprivation and psychopathology (Minuchin et al., 1967; Riessman, Cohen, and Pearl, 1964). Recent scientific literature presents further evidence of the relationship between family and individual mental health. Harvey and Bray (1991), for example, found that stressful life events, including relational patterns between parents and siblings, were related to increased levels of psychological distress and mental illness. Voydanoff and Donnelly (1989) also determined that unemployment, instability, uncertainty, and economic difficulties invariably lead to severe family and personal stresses. A strong connection has been found between parental distress and children's behavioral problems (Meyer, 1995; Sharlin and Elshansky, 1997). Moreover, it has also been documented that personal distress and estrangement have a strong, negative impact on family functioning (Anderson, 1992; Dumas and Wekerle, 1995). Hence emerges the pattern of the vicious cycle, with different family problems affecting one another in a circular movement.

Criminal Behavior and Drug Abuse

Scientific evidence suggests that impaired parenting and family relationships are determining variables in the development of criminal behavior (Farrington, 1990; Henggeler et al., 1991; Minuchin et al., 1967; Patterson and Bank, 1986; Sampson and Laub, 1994; Tolan and Loeber, 1993). Gorman-Smith (1996) examined the relationship between family patterns and participation in violent and nonviolent delinquent behavior among inner-city minority youths. They concluded that youngsters who developed violent behavior grew up with very little discipline, cohesion, or involvement in their families. Other researchers have also initiated studies on the influence of the family on the development of criminal behavior (Kuperminc and Repucci, 1996; McCord, 1996; Tolan and Loeber, 1993). According to McCord (1996), the family is the best predictor for the development of delinquent behavior: "Family interaction and socialization practices contribute to the causes of violence" (p. 147). Tolan and Loeber (1993) found that "erratic, threatening and harsh discipline, low supervision and a shaky parent-child attachment mediate the effects of poverty and other structural factors or discipline" (p. 523).

A similar connection exists between family patterns and drug abuse. Extensive evidence points to the negative influence that drug-addicted parents have on their children (Famularo, Kinscherff, and Fenton, 1992; Gawin and Ellinwood, 1988). Naturally, we can expect adolescents exposed to drugs in their homes to be more likely to become addicts themselves. There is proof that children's interactions with their parents are a major determinant in the development of pathological behavior, including drug abuse (Andrews et al., 1993; Patterson, 1972; Patterson and Bank, 1989). Furthermore, a new direction in research suggests that "siblings appear to contribute to the adolescent's subsequent substance use" (Duncan, 1996, p. 158).

Child Care, Child Development, and the Multiproblem Family

Although in the 1970s a great deal of attention was given to parental functioning, in the 1980s and 1990s, the focus was directed toward the children. Some evidence suggests that severe poverty is strongly related to the cognitive and emotional development of children (Bernstein, 1960, 1961, 1962, 1964; Brodley, 1989; Deutch, 1963, 1965; Duncan, Brooks-Gunn, and Klebanov, 1994; McLoyd, 1989, 1990; Patterson, Crosby, and Vuchinich, 1992; Rutter, 1981). It is no wonder that children growing up in severe economic deprivation are exposed, from birth, to "harsh discipline, lack of maternal warmth, exposure to aggressive adult models, maternal aggressive values, family life stressors, mother's lack of social support, peer group instability, and lack of stimulation" (Dodge, Pettit, and Bates, 1994).

According to Kaslow (1995), the premise adopted by most cultures, from biblical days to the present, is that the family's primary function is to bear and raise children. However, even though most multiproblem families have numerous children, they pay little attention, if any, to raising them. Most of these children are born either out of wedlock or as a result of unwanted pregnancies. The mothers receive no prenatal care or guidance, and the newborns' nutrition and medical attention are well below standard (Tarnowski and Rohrbeck, 1993). These children, therefore, are at an above-average risk of developing complications at birth or serious illnesses during the first years of their lives (Kaslow, 1995; Needleman et al., 1990; Rivara and Mueller, 1987). They grow up in crime-ridden communities, overcrowded housing, unsanitary conditions, and, all too often, with alcoholic or drug-addicted parents. In short, these children are unwanted children raised by unfit parents. They are neglected by parents who do not wish to invest any energy or other resources in the already difficult task of raising them. As Kaslow states, "These addictions and extreme squander of the family's financial resources, if they have them, consume inordinate amounts of time and energy, diverting them from their spousal and parenting roles, and contributing to their acting in inappropriate, ineffective, and often damaging ways" (Kaslow, 1995, p. 171).

In addition, the parents, living in constant distress and despair, tend to take out their frustrations on the children by abusing them physically, emotionally, and, in severe cases, even sexually. Conger and Conger (1994), for instance, report that "High levels of spousal irritability with coercive exchanges over money matters were expected to be associated with greater hostility towards the children. . . . Overall results were consistent with the proposed model" (p. 54). In the face of constant criticism and humiliation, these children do not develop any sense of security or self-confidence. They grow up, from the very beginning, feeling unmotivated and hopeless, and, in many cases, their situation does not improve when they become adults and parents themselves. As a result, they end up neglecting and abusing their own children as well, thereby repeating the vicious cycle of child neglect.

In sum, during the early years, literature about multiproblem families was based largely on casework and clinical work, whereas recently it has become much more common to conduct qualitative or quantitative empirical studies. However, despite extensive clinical experience and voluminous research on the consequences of poverty for children and adolescents, as well as on its relationship to parenthood, mental health, delinquency, and drug abuse, little attention has been given to the spouses and the relationship between them. The spousal dyad serves as the core; the most important subsystem in the development of the entire family system, functioning as the source of the family's health and welfare.

It seems to us that by overlooking the spousal subsystem, we are missing critical knowledge and understanding of the multiproblem family phenomenon. We believe in the notion that "People of all ages can best develop their lives and be enhanced by remaining with . . . or relying on, their family as an important resource of support" (Ronnau and Marlow, 1993, p. 540). We estimate, therefore, that to fully understand the complexity of the multiple-problem family and to provide them with adequate help, we have the responsibility of continuing research. It is not enough to understand that poverty and disorganization may lead to drug addiction; we need to comprehend the different factors affecting the family and how they interact. The family is an integral unit, and anything affecting it in one part will inevitably bring about reactions in other parts, a fact that reinforces the need to deal with the family as a whole.

Multiproblem families live in deep economic deprivation, in addition to a plethora of other problems. Their perpetual distress and despair is inevitably transmitted from generation to generation. That is why we choose to call them "families in extreme distress" (FED). We believe that this concept best expresses, not only the continuity and multiplicity of problems, but also the difficult emotional condition in which these families try to survive. We shall now proceed to review different attempts at clinical intervention with FED.

Chapter 2

The Hope: Clinical Interventions with Families in Extreme Distress

As described in the previous chapter, the phenomenon of families in extreme distress has been in existence for a very long time, as have ongoing attempts to deal with it. Intervention with this population began after World War II and continued until the worldwide economic crisis at the beginning of the 1970s. All meaningful resources for intervention projects with poor and unorganized families started to be eliminated, and by the late 1970s, one could hardly find any projects concerning intervention with such families (Lorion, 1978). In addition to the financial aspect of decreasing intervention efforts, another contributing factor was probably the overpowering atmosphere of despair and difficulty that emerged when working with FED.

In examining the different intervention approaches, Lorion (1973, 1978) focused on four major topics that determined the reluctance of many therapists to undertake interventions with families in extreme distress. The first topic refers to the discrepancy between the FED and the availability of adequate services. The second topic focuses on the inconsistency in treatment acceptance, attrition, and varying outcomes, which consequently prevent a clear-cut presentation of effective results—a must for obtaining the necessary financial resources in the atmosphere of economic restraint that has prevailed over the past twenty-five years in Western societies. The third topic deals with the attitudes of FED, often based on cultural and socioeconomic diversity, as well as their expectations from treatment, which are quite different from those of professionals. Finally, the fourth topic refers to the therapists' attitudes and their expectations for successful outcomes from intervention with FED. Frequent disappointment with results has caused avoidance behavior when being "forced" to work with FED.

Fortunately, not all clinicians avoid intervention with FED. Some clinicians even perceive such treatment as a mission, either personal or professional. As a result, we find remarkable efforts in trying to help FED during the past five decades. Since intervention with FED is very complex and requires examination of family and community systems on different levels (behavioral, cognitive, emotional), it is important to understand that no single method of intervention can be prescribed, while emphasizing the need to be familiar with the character, content, and structure of past and present experiences. Each experience adds another piece to the intricate puzzle that constitutes the treatment of FED.

HISTORICAL REVIEW: INTERVENTION WITH MULTIPLE-PROBLEM FAMILIES

The 1900s Through the 1960s

The earliest interventions with poor families were undertaken at the beginning of the century by the "friendly visitors," founders of the social work profession. They chose to live in poor neighborhoods, and their intervention was based on resocialization of poor families. The friendly visitor taught the family what to do by guiding and advising from a position of superiority. Most of their activities were not based on solid professional knowledge, but rather on a spiritual commitment to improve society by helping the poor. As much as this kind of intervention would be dismissed today, it should be examined in the context of the period, as one cannot ignore its pioneering contribution. The current work of professional social workers is rooted in the efforts and commitment of those friendly visitors. Historically, the social workers' obligation has always been toward poor and disadvantaged families. This obligation was somewhat weakened by the strong impact of psychoanalysis and its effect on social work and casework. The desire to increase professional knowledge and performance encouraged social workers to utilize psychodynamic concepts and techniques, which did not necessarily serve the needs of those families (Geismar and La Sorte, 1964). Even Freud (1950) recognized that dynamically oriented approaches to treatment would have to be modified to take into consideration the reality and lifestyle of the poor. However, many social work agencies proceeded toward specialization and service fragmentation to enable the implementation of psychodynamic concepts. Eventually, the diminishing influence of these theories shifted social work perceptions back to "external" reality as having a meaningful impact on working with disadvantaged families. Since then, more attempts have been made to help this population, although most of them were not evaluated until Geismar and La Sorte (1964) created a taxonomy to organize these efforts according to the approaches used in treatment, as follows:

1. The intensive casework approach is based on conventional techniques used in social casework, sometimes allied with a more assertive approach, such as frequent home visits. A casework approach includes diagnosis and treatment of the entire family by the social worker, as well as coordination of various other available services. Most of the intensive casework done up to the end of the 1960s was dominated by a psychodynamic orientation, as a result of the education that most social workers had acquired (Kaplan, 1984).
2. The case conference approach is based on presenting a case by various workers from a formally assembled group. The group presents its diagnosis and treatment plan and assigns responsibility for the treatment to one or more workers within one or more agencies. In the absence of one designated person to organize the plan, this approach has not proven to be very effective for multiproblem families. It has, however, been widely used among social workers when intervening with difficult and hard-to-reach families. With this approach, the range of problems can be so overwhelming that it pushes the social worker to delegate intervention tasks rather than taking into account the special character of the family, which calls for one person to take charge in helping the family to get organized (Geismar and La Sorte, 1964).
3. The multiservice approach involves the consolidation of treatments administered by different organizations in various areas of specialization, while a totally separate organization is re-

sponsible for the coordination of the treatment approaches (Geismar and La Sorte, 1964). Due to the discrepancy between services that may require clients to perform numerous and often conflicting tasks, this approach may have an overwhelmingly negative impact on the family. It should be noted that coordinating treatments does not guarantee supervision of all the details that make up a treatment approach.

4. The community development approach refers to programs that are aimed at strengthening the entire community as a context for the individual family unit. These programs include a variety of services, such as full-day and after-school child care, parents' groups, and support groups to prevent adolescents from becoming involved in delinquency and drug abuse. It is important to note that many of the social service programs developed in the 1960s centered around the community development approach.
5. Other approaches incorporate the community development approach while taking into account the individual family. Accordingly, a volunteer to guide the family or a professional who works together with the parents (especially the mothers) is sent by the community service agency to individual families as needed.

According to Schlesinger (1970) and Kaplan (1984), the previous categories remain valid even after twenty years.

The most influential project of this period was the Family Centered Project of St. Paul, Minnesota (Birt, 1956; Compton, 1962, 1979). The project was undertaken between 1947 and 1968 by agencies in St. Paul and was aimed at improving treatment for poor and unorganized families. The idea to develop this project arose from a survey indicating that 6 percent of families accounted for 50 percent of social services used in the city of St. Paul. Despite the enormous amount of energy invested in working with each family, usually long term, the treatment was fragmented, crisis oriented, and symptomatically focused. The project had four main goals: (1) to provide in-home service to hard-to-reach and resistant families, (2) to focus on the entire family rather than on the individual, (3) to build a collaborative work attitude with the family by reaching mutually agreed-upon therapeutic goals, and (4) to work toward strengthening the family. An innovative aspect of the project was that one worker retained primary responsibility for the family and coordinated the various community resources needed by the family.

A decade later, in 1979, Compton criticized the project for lacking a theoretical framework. She emphasized the essence of worker-family collaboration in creating change and the importance of building a sense of family strength and competence. She strongly recommended that direct service and community support be given concomitantly. She objected to brief programs for multiproblem families, pointing out that families who have a history of personal defeat and negative experiences with social services need the time to build up trust and should therefore be given intensive long-term treatment.

A project similar to the St. Paul Family Centered Project was the New Haven Neighborhood Improvement Project (NIP), which was conducted in the early 1960s. It was undertaken at Farnum Courts, a small, low-income housing project in New Haven, Connecticut, which is mostly populated by immigrants of various ethnic backgrounds. The project included intensive work with hard-to-reach cases, as well as group work within the community. The project was evaluated by Geismar (Geismar and Krisberg, 1967), who was deeply involved in the St. Paul project. The outcome revealed two main issues relevant to the development of intervention with this population.

The first issue refers to the emphasis on community organization, which was to become one of the dominant tools used by social workers and other mental health professionals in the 1960s and early 1970s (Alexander, 1973; Billingsley, 1969; Geismar, 1971b; Riessman, 1967; Woodbury and Woodbury, 1969). Despite the efforts of Geismar and Krisberg (1967) to underscore the absence of data that might indicate the importance of community organization to the overall improvement of the families who had participated in the NIP, social workers were inspired by the possibility of reaching entire communities rather than just individuals or families. They were sure that by using the community approach, services would become available to a larger population, and, at the same time, the level of accountability would be raised. Community intervention seemed more promising than the intensive, often hopeless, work with a few hard-to-reach families. In contrast to this unbridled enthusiasm, Meyer (1963) points out that the only shared characteristic of multiproblem families is poverty and that all other problems are specific to each family. Thus, without ignoring the importance of community networks, basic needs of these families appear to have been overlooked. The second issue refers to the length of the NIP intervention. Although severely disorganized families underwent intensive casework for a minimum of eighteen months, the greatest and most meaningful changes were achieved in the first six months of treatment.

The tendency to approach multiproblem families through community intervention paralleled the development of systemic thinking within psychotherapy, which is the core theory of family therapy, as opposed to that of individual psychodynamic casework. Accordingly, we find interesting attempts to intervene with and treat the entire family, rather than focusing on individual members (Chilman, 1966; Levine, 1964; Meyer, 1963; Minuchin and Montalvo, 1968; Minuchin et al., 1967; Woodbury and Woodbury, 1969).

Undoubtedly, the work of Minuchin and his colleagues (Minuchin and Montalvo, 1968; Minuchin et al., 1967) at the Wiltwyck School for Boys had a very meaningful effect on the field of multiproblem family intervention. Minuchin and his colleagues conducted a study of twelve families with more than one juvenile delinquent. Treatment was provided to the entire family, as well as to subsystems of the family (parents and siblings). The study recommended working with the family as a system, while recognizing family strengths rather than pathology. The main focus of treatment was the structuring of boundaries, leadership, and rules by acknowledging the family's ability to form an organized system.

We can view the two and a half decades from the end of World War II through the late 1960s as a period of meaningful change in attitudes toward poor and disorganized families. These changes affected the direction of a large number of projects and studies conducted by various mental health centers and social welfare agencies. The absence of theoretical and practical knowledge was replaced by the enthusiasm of the "pioneers": the social workers, community workers, psychiatrists, counselors, and even "nonprofessionals" who tried to work with distressed families in hopes of helping them (Pearl and Riessman, 1965; Riessman, 1967).

The 1970s

The 1970s brought about meaningful changes in dealing with the phenomenon of poor and distressed families. There was hope, enthusiasm, and commitment to working with this population, spurred by the humanitarian spirit of the West after World War II. However, the opposite trend, rooted in the world economic crisis, left the issue of families in extreme distress and their needs without adequate solutions. Budget cuts mostly affected the weaker population, including poor, unorganized, and distressed families. The decision to drastically cut services was based on results from different projects carried out in the 1960s, which had the somewhat naive goals of completely changing the poverty-culture lifestyle and preventing the phenomenon of multiproblem families. Thus, the literature of the 1970s on interventions with poor populations describes, analyzes, and develops strategies based on low-cost budgets.

Although family therapy flourished and acquired experience and a deeper understanding by working with different kinds of families, it seemed that poor, disorganized families were not attractive clients. Yet, some professionals still did not give up. One of them was Harry J. Aponte, who followed Minuchin in the Philadelphia Child Guidance Clinic and has been practicing since the 1970s and into the present (Aponte, 1974a, 1974b, 1976a, 1976b, 1979a, 1979b, 1982, 1985a, 1985b, 1986, 1989, 1990, 1991, 1994). Aponte (1976a) defined multiproblem families as "underorganized families" rather than disorganized families, a term that was used by Minuchin and associates (1967). The term underorganized families refers to the lack of organization rather than chaotic organization. Lack of organization is defined as a structure that has never developed, therefore leaving the family without a sense of identity, stability, and flexibility. Underorganization, according to Aponte, is an ecosystem phenomenon. It develops within specific communities that have become, in some ways, the scapegoats of society. The norms, values, and morals of society at large, which are usually propagated by institutions, are therefore not acceptable in these communities.

In dealing with underorganized families, Aponte recommends intervention on two levels. On one level, he relates to the family's internal organization and uses structural techniques similar to those of Minuchin (1974). These techniques involve joining with the family's pain, distress, and hopelessness and helping them to strengthen their ability to survive under difficult conditions by providing the stimulus to build basic organizational skills within the family. The other level relates to the dynamics of the relationships between the family and its everyday contacts. The ecostructural approach defines the different systems with which the family interacts. Assessment is based on the type of interactions and their effect and importance in relation to the functioning of the family. It is recommended to begin intervention with the system that has the strongest influence on the family. In many of his case illustrations, Aponte describes work focused on the children's relationship with the educational system (e.g., Aponte, 1974a, 1976b). Although not specifically mentioned, it seems that one way to join the distress of those families is by following through with the parents' commitment to their children (Gatti and Colman, 1976; Goldstein, 1973; Jones, Neuman, and Shyne, 1976; Maybanks and Bryce, 1979).

The ecosystem approach follows the 1960s' concept of social contacts, especially those with the immediate community and social institutions. The ecological approach highlights the weakness of linear thinking, often used when planning community organization strategies and interventions. Linear thinking suggests a problem-solving approach, meaning that a specific problem is addressed by a specific service. However, it does not take into consideration the resistance of disadvantaged populations to social institutions and their inability to use social services. When planning services for multiproblem families, a holistic approach must be considered, which will include constant interaction between the different services, as well as between the families and the services (Argles and MacKenzie, 1970; Auerwald, 1972; Burt, 1976a, 1976b; Mazer, 1972; Schiff and Kalter, 1980).

An example of this approach is the Nashville Comprehensive Emergency Services Project, which coordinated services for abused and neglected children (Burt, 1976a, 1976b). When planning the program, special attention was given to the interaction between the different emergency services provided, such as emergency shelters, emergency caretakers, and home services. The results of this program show an impressive decrease in the number of children removed from their families. This project is a typical example of the attempts at working with multiproblem families in the 1970s. It offers an ecological approach designed to help children with their own family's committed involvement. Another component is the "emergency" type of service, which reflects the trend toward meaningful brief interventions in the 1970s, in general, and interventions with multiproblem families, in particular.

The development of the brief, short-term type of intervention was influenced by substantial budget cuts in social and mental health services and by severe criticism of long-term, often psychodynamic, interventions (Eysenck, 1952) and research results, thus indicating that short-term therapy can be as effective as long-term therapy (Shlein, Mosak, and Dreikurs, 1962; Butcher and Ross, 1978). In the area of family therapy, the 1970s reveal many creative approaches that have enriched the field, most of them brief, short term, and focused. They are defined as the "strategic approach," "the Milan approach," or "the solution-focused approach" and have been the leading techniques in family therapy for more than two decades (Boscolo et al., 1987; de Shazer, 1985; Haley, 1976; Madanes, 1981; O'Hanlon and Weiner-Davis, 1989; Papp, 1983; Selvini-Palazzoli et al., 1978; Watzlawick, Weakland, and Fisch, 1974).

These changes, along with Lorion's (1974) findings, which show that brief therapies may be particularly effective in cases dealing with populations from the lower socioeconomic or educational strata, opened up a new direction for intervention with multiproblem families. The brief and focused approach is centered around problem solving, either by defining the problem and its impact on the entire family system (Boscolo et al., 1987; Haley, 1976; Watzlawick, Weakland, and Fisch, 1974) or by defining the expected solution (de Shazer, 1985; O'Hanlon and Weiner-Davis, 1989). When either the problem or the solution are defined, various techniques are then employed, including reframing, paradox, tasks, rituals, developing communication skills, and more. The brief intervention method is time limited, concentrating on a specific goal and requiring active participation by the therapist. All of these ingredients are needed when working with multiproblem families because of their difficulty in committing to long-term, abstract interventions. Sometimes their hopelessness is expressed in their passive attitude, requiring active involvement on the part of the therapist to overcome the attitude and push the family toward change (Aronson, 1966). Positive results, as well as client satisfaction, have been reported in many cases of brief therapy (Alexander and Parsons, 1973; Bulehorn, 1978; Cade, 1975; Parsons and Alexander, 1973; Yamamoto and Goin, 1966). Most of these interventions were focused on specific areas that were usually connected to parenting and children's issues. Combining brief therapy with family therapy has proven to be an effective strategy with multiproblem families (Jones, Neuman, and Shyne, 1976; Mostwin, 1980; Rosenthal et al., 1974).

The last half of the 1970s has defined the new direction in intervening with multiproblem families. Instead of large community projects, the interventions have been more modest, focusing on a specific, well-defined problem within a particular time frame, while taking into consideration the entire family system and its relation to the immediate ecological context. Undoubtedly, even if the trend leads to more effective outcomes, the difficulties of working with multiproblem families, along with the job's low prestige and diminished financial resources, have reduced the number of therapists committed to helping this population.

The 1980s and 1990s

The 1980s and 1990s have been characterized by a relatively small number of intervention attempts with the poor and multiproblem population. However, at the same time, more efforts have been made to find out why it is so difficult and frustrating to work with this population. As a way to overcome the frustration, therapists and clients have tended to favor the joint-goal intervention approach. This is carried out mostly in the home, where therapists delegate authority as a means of strengthening and preserving the family unit through empowerment. These family strengthening and family preservation programs have become the main treatment approach of the 1980s and 1990s.

Let us first try to understand the frustration in such therapeutic interaction. For many years, multiproblem families were described as "hard-to-reach" or "unmotivated" clients. Working with them was labeled as unstructured, fragmented, and interminable, usually without positive results. Therefore, it is not surprising to find that many clinicians ignored this population. Furthermore, the sharply reduced financial resources and the sparse attention allocated to this population created a low-prestige image among professionals. It was more attractive to develop theoretical and practical expertise in more "glorified" fields. Those who remained committed to multiproblem families applied intervention techniques related to specific issues such as child abuse in poor and unorganized families. Most of them concentrated on preventing the removal of children from their homes to foster families or to institutions. Therapists found that, in many of the cases, home-based services, which included family and parental counseling, succeeded in obtaining parental cooperation and resulted in subsequent improvement in parents' child-rearing methods (Compler, 1983; Heying, 1985; Magura, 1981; McGowan and Meesan, 1983; Munroe-Blum, Boyle, and Offord, 1988; Shaw et al., 1994; Skurray and Ham, 1990).

Special attention has also been given to variables connected with immigration and the wide variety of needs expressed by different cultural backgrounds that, in many cases, may contribute to the creation of poverty and disorganization (Aponte, 1993; Boyd-Franklin, 1989; Garcia-Preto, 1982). Analysis of these issues emphasizes cooperation and the creation of dialogue, as well as a search for family strengths and resilience (Kim-Berg, 1991; Saleebey, 1992; Wang and Gordon, 1994; Wolin and Wolin, 1993). This emphasis on family strength and resilience in interventions with poor and disorganized families is based on recognizing their ability to survive under difficult and often hopeless conditions. Overlooking certain basic moral rules, one must acknowledge the creativity demonstrated by these families in their everyday survival efforts. Thus, if we regard certain antisocial behavior as necessary for survival, then we must reverse our attitude toward the family and allow for a respectful dialogue between client and therapist.

Accepting this philosophy leads us to conclude that the family has its strengths and that therapy should not only concentrate on teaching problem-solving skills but also create therapeutic situations wherein the family can experience their strengths and resilience, mainly through empowerment (Saleebey, 1992; Wang and Gordon, 1994; Wolin and Wolin, 1993). This philosophy is the basis for family preservation programs,* whose primary assumption is that the best way to help children is through strengthening and empowering the family as a unit. Removing the child from the family is a traumatic experience for the child and the family, even if child neglect or abuse is present. It is strongly believed that strengthening and empowering both parents and the parent-child subsystem enables the family to develop adequate resilience and competence to effectively control their lives. Family preservation programs are usually designed to include cooperation between family and community-environment resources (Aponte, 1994; Brossman, 1990; Bryce and Lloyd, 1981; Kaplan, 1986; Kim-Berg, 1991; Whitaker et al., 1990). In addition to the variety of family preservation projects, some common practice principles are followed, such as providing services to the family as a unit and working together as a team, thereby eliminating the need for referral to different therapists, counselors, and/or social workers who hardly communicate among themselves.

Intervention includes family therapy, which is usually time limited, focused, and goal oriented. Goals and procedures are decided upon jointly by the therapeutic team and the family. In addition to the actual family treatment, special attention is given to the cooperation between the family and relevant institutions and resources in the community (Aponte, 1994; Kim-Berg, 1991). It is important to differentiate between in-home treatment, which is similar to home visits, and the home-based treatment provided by family preservation programs. In-home treatment sessions are usually held at home, for practical reasons, mainly because the family cannot organize the time or make the commitment to come to the therapist's office. The family preservation program, in contrast, provides home-based treatment based on the philosophy of respect toward family issues and toward being part of a family, home, and community (Aponte, 1994).

---

*Family preservation programs are often called home-based services/treatment or in-home treatment.

When summarizing the development of intervention with multiproblem families, it is surprising to note that many basic elements of intervention had already been suggested in the 1950s and 1960s. However, experience has enriched these basic technical aspects of intervention, clearly evident in the family preservation programs that have become the main venue for intervention during the 1980s and 1990s. These programs are based on integrating community intervention, widely used in the 1960s and the early 1970s, with family intervention as a unit, also recognized in the 1960s and further developed in the 1970s. The programs incorporate the brief therapy techniques that were the main focus of the late 1970s. Another trend that started in the 1960s devoted a great deal of attention to children and parenting.

The most important change appears to have occurred in the attitude toward helping poor and unorganized families. The naive notion of the 1950s and 1960s persuaded many professionals that the "war against poverty" could be resolved with adequate resources, especially financial ones. Gradually, a more mature understanding has evolved, showing the need for realistic expectations regarding interventions with disadvantaged families. Special emphasis is placed on the recognition and respect shown to families for their decisions and for every small improvement in their problem-solving skills, while at the same time acknowledging the therapists' difficulties and their level of frustration. This insight may be effectively used in reshaping intervention plans for multiproblem populations.

APPROACHES, TECHNIQUES, AND PRINCIPLES OF INTERVENTION WITH FED

Based on past experience, we find that it is possible to formulate effective policies and directions for therapeutic intervention with poor and multiproblem families. Such policies must set forth the type of intervention, the place of intervention, the methods used by therapists, and the type of therapist-family relationship.

Type of Intervention with FED

The type of intervention suggests two important dimensions: (1) the focus on multilevel intervention, including the family and/or the community, and (2) the principles guiding the type of intervention.

Regarding the first dimension, the focus of intervention, we learn from past experience with FED that limited intervention can offer remedies on one level only, either at the individual, the family, or the community level, thus leaving many FED issues without adequate recourse. Consequently, even if a particular short-term intervention were to be effective, the family could still remain frustrated and mistrusting of social services, and, eventually, even positive results of the intervention could be lost. This highlights the need to structure a multilevel intervention approach that focuses on the individual and the family, as well as on community services.

Multilevel intervention has been practiced in various forms since the 1940s, acknowledging the futility of any approach that does not take into account the complexity of FED. More recently, the approach has been named "the ecostructural approach" (Aponte, 1994) or "family preservation" (Kim-Berg, 1991). It involves intensive family therapy with a simultaneous attempt at building a supportive community network with appropriate social services. It focuses on the family as the framework within which to deal with issues related to child-rearing difficulties, parenthood, marriage, or adult functioning problems. It further emphasizes the importance of ongoing relations between the family and community services in dealing with matters such as school problems, employment, and medical services. The approach also stresses the need for developing community services that would be responsive to the needs of the poor, unorganized families and individuals.

Multilevel intervention, although not always fully implemented, has been recognized as important by many of those who have dealt with the FED population (Aponte, 1976a, 1994; Birt, 1956; Compton, 1962, 1979; Geismar and Krisberg, 1967; Geismar and La Sorte, 1964; Minuchin, 1970). It has often been criticized when failing to include the larger context of FED within a program, namely, the individual, the family, community services, and their interactions.

On the second important dimension, dealing with the principles guiding the type of intervention, it has been previously mentioned that most intervention approaches, through the end of the 1960s, were dominated by a psychodynamic orientation. This was a result of the education acquired by the majority of mental health professionals (Kaplan, 1984). Although one cannot ignore the effective elements of a psychodynamic orientation in relation to FED, such as extended concern and support, other aspects of its principles and techniques are not sufficient when intervening with FED. One technique common to this orientation focuses on the interpsychic level, but as most FED are overwhelmed by their interpersonal difficulties, this method is hardly effective with the FED population. On the other hand, the benefits and effectiveness of structured therapy have been clearly demonstrated (de Shazer, 1985; Haley, 1976; Minuchin et al., 1967; Minuchin, 1974; Minuchin and Fishman, 1981) with the therapist playing an active role and proposing a focused goal with time limits.

Structured intervention is basic in effective work with FED (Minuchin and Montalvo, 1968; Minuchin et al., 1967). Structuring means establishing a well-defined contract with the family concerning the goal of therapy, the issues that will be dealt with in the process, the duration of treatment sessions, and a definition of the therapist's and the client's responsibilities. Structuring provides many families with their first basis for organization, seeing that most of them are characterized as either chaotic (Minuchin et al., 1967) or lacking organization altogether (Aponte, 1976a). Within structured intervention, there is room for different kinds of therapeutic approaches that are related to the defined goal. One such approach is that of structured family therapy, with its emphasis on clear boundaries between subsystems within the family, as well as between the family and the outside world, and a clear definition of family hierarchy roles and rules (Aponte, 1994; Minuchin et al., 1967). Another approach is that of problem solving (Kim-Berg, 1991), which concentrates on specific issues usually chosen by the family. Structured intervention is concerned with the question of time as well, that is, how long the intervention will last. The duration of interventions with FED has long been debated among professionals. Some experts have demonstrated the effectiveness and adaptability of brief therapies for FED (Alexander and Parsons, 1973; Bulehorn, 1978; Jones, Neuman, and Shyne, 1976; Parsons and Alexander, 1973; Rosenthal et al., 1974; Yamamoto and Goin, 1966), citing such benefits as a reduction in their frustration level and the opportunity to experience some sense of success in a relatively short period of time. Others have criticized brief therapy (Compton, 1979), claiming that the families need more time to build the trust and confidence necessary to begin work on their severe difficulties. Minuchin (1970) recognized the need for long-term intervention with multiproblem families, but pointed out that combining family intervention with community support systems might reduce the duration of such treatment. This clearly indicates the need to adopt a multilevel intervention approach to FED.

Place of Intervention

Home-based intervention has been found to be very effective in working with FED (Aponte, 1991; Kim-Berg, 1991; Rabin, Rosenbaum, and Sens, 1982; Sharlin, Shamai, and Gilad-Smolinsky, 1994; Tavantzis et al., 1985). Organizing therapeutic sessions within the family territory, its home, is seen as filling a practical need, as well as respecting the "belonging" atmosphere of the family. Setting up therapeutic sessions at home eases the logistical aspects of intervention, since for many FED, getting all family members together at a specific time and place seems to be nearly an impossible task. Accepting the fact that FED find it very difficult to arrive at a designated social service location for repeated therapeutic sessions raises the issue of reaching out to them rather than just waiting until they come for help. The care and concern that is demonstrated toward the family by the therapists' repeated home visits adds to the family's basic trust in social services and their agents.

The Therapist System

One difficult challenge when working with FED is that oftentimes the therapist has feelings of despair similar to those of the family (Shamai and Sharlin, 1996). As early as the 1950s, Geismar and La Sorte (1964) recognized the need for more than one therapist and coined it "the conference approach." Whereas this approach is based on assembling the therapists' team for diagnostic purposes only, later approaches have regarded the therapeutic team as the implementer of the entire process (Compler, 1983; Rabin, 1989;

Sharlin and Shamai, 1995). Rabin (1989) suggested that the team should consist of a male and a female therapist who enter the family with equal authority and become role models for effective ways of communication for the entire family.

Another perspective of teamwork is described by Compler (1983), who refers to the team working with the family as an "interagency team." This team has three clearly defined and essential roles: (1) case manager, (2) clinical social worker or family therapist, and (3) paraprofessional and family aide, when needed. Compler (1983) specifies that the interagency team is characterized by an ongoing relationship between the case manager and family therapist, over a period of some months, in the development of joint therapeutic goals together with the family. Their cooperation involves team discussions in the form of a case conference on operating procedures, values, services, activities, and therapeutic changes in their clients. However, Compler (1983) does not indicate whether both the case manager and family therapist should be present at the same, or at separate, therapy sessions.

Considering the specific character of FED, clearly, the family therapist needs to work in conjunction with the case manager in initiating, implementing and supporting the family's efforts to connect with the environment. All of this cannot be accomplished by a single person. It is also very important for the family to identify the role of the case manager as a resource coordinator and as the representative of an agency, separate from the role of the therapist. This distinction allows the therapist to continue working with the family even when its members are disappointed about their failure to gain access to a particular community resource. It also provides a positive model for the family in terms of role distribution and definition.

The model previously described by Sharlin and Shamai (1995), as well as that presented later in this book, follows Compler (1983), with the family therapist and case manager having defined and distinctive, yet interacting, roles. Both therapist and case manager are present in the therapeutic sessions. This strategy generates a model of communication on contradictory issues, problem solving, and negotiation.

Type of Therapist-Client Relationship

The therapist-client relationship within the field of family therapy has undergone meaningful changes. The pioneers of family therapy contradict classical psychoanalytical approaches by creating a setting in which they are very active, often giving directions and assigning concrete tasks (de Shazer, 1985; Haley, 1976; Madanes, 1981; Minuchin, 1974; Minuchin and Fishman, 1981; O'Hanlon and Weiner-Davis, 1989; Watzlawick, Weakland, and Fisch, 1974). Followers, such as social constructionists, stressed the role of the therapist in enabling dialogue that empowers the family in finding strength to deal with its difficulties (Kim-Berg, 1991; McNamee and Gergen, 1992).

The complexity of FED requires integrating both trends to empower the family to seek its strengths, to develop a sense of potency, and to believe in itself. This must be done through active leadership on the part of the therapeutic team, which challenges and directs the family. It does not mean taking a patronizing position, but rather having a dialogue in which the therapist shares his or her own knowledge and experience with the family, thereby enriching its repertoire of strength.

Experience has shown the strength of poor, disorganized families can be explored and activated through multilevel intervention. Such therapy should be performed by a team with defined roles and the means to develop a dialogue with the family in a structured context, using the family home as a base for implementing intervention.

PART II: FROM THEORY TO PRACTICE— AN OVERVIEW OF THE MODEL

Chapter 3

The Fear of Working with FED: Overcoming the Coalition of Despair

Working with families in extreme distress is often not very appealing to mental health professionals, including social workers who, ideologically, should be committed to this population (Lorion, 1978; Shamai and Sharlin, 1996). It is not easy to discover the reasons for these reservations, as they are often expressed indirectly. This can be accomplished, however, by attaching young and inexperienced physicians and therapists to these clients (Lorion, 1978) or by raising "as if" professional questions, such as "Why work with the entire family and not with each individual, since person-to-person intervention might touch on a 'deeper' level?"; "Why not work only with the children, if there is a better chance for changes with the younger generation?"; "if the fathers in these families do not have any influence, nor do they want to be involved in treatment, would it be more useful to support and strengthen only the mothers?"

Professionals who dare express some of their hidden thoughts usually indicate that working with some of these families is always ineffective and might be a waste of time and energy. However, since they are under the "responsibility" of an institution (it can be a mental health clinic, a social services department, or just a general hospital), one cannot ignore these families. Some professionals maintain that only a minimal amount of energy should be focused on this population, and only in cases of acute crises. For many, working with poor and distressed families is not considered a subject of expertise. Working with FED is considered generic, low-prestige work that "must be done," thus increasing the possibilities for worker burnout.

When analyzing twenty social workers' reports about families in extreme distress and adding these to direct dialogue with these workers, we observed a phenomenon, which we named "coalition of despair" between social workers and FED (Shamai and Sharlin, 1996). The phenomenon is characterized by a startling symmetry of attitudes, feelings, and behaviors shared by social workers and families in extreme distress. The outcome of this coalition is that social workers and other helping professionals experience diminished confidence in their capability to work with distressed families. It creates fear, which either prevents or limits creativity and the desire to invest in the complicated process of intervention with families in extreme distress. Thus, part of these "professional questions" related to the efficiency of working with families in extreme distress were rooted in the fear of failure, burnout, or despair, familiar emotions to those who had either intervened with families in distress or had learned about such interventions. Although we observed the phenomenon of the coalition of despair among social workers, similar manifestations can be seen among other helping professionals when working with FED (Lorion, 1978).

THE COALITION OF DESPAIR

The coalition of despair comes into being when social workers' and families' attitudes and behaviors converge. Polansky (1965, 1971; Polansky, Borgman, and DeSaix, 1972; Polansky, DeSaix, and Sharlin, 1972) points to a similar phenomenon in communication between social workers and clients, calling it "verbal inaccessibility." Polansky discovered that social workers who spend long periods treating verbally inaccessible clients tend to imitate their behavior and become verbally inaccessible themselves. The contamination goes beyond mere speechlessness. The cognitive and behavioral malfunctioning of these families is also adopted by social workers in their interventions with this population. Workers may exhibit characteristics such as disorganization, lack of boundaries, poor verbal ability, concrete thinking, low frustration tolerance, and aggressiveness. As a result, they experience pseudohelplessness and feel powerless to reduce the pain for which the families sought help. Four areas seem to be critical in creating the coalition of despair: disorganization and lack of boundaries, thinking and language patterns, frustration and aggression, and hopelessness and helplessness.

Disorganization and Lack of Boundaries

Disorganization implies a lack of boundaries, resulting in vague definition of roles, poor sense of time, and lack of consistency. A number of studies indicate that disorganization is a principal feature among these families (Aponte, 1976a, 1976b; Dax and Hagger, 1977; Long and Vaillant, 1984; Minuchin et al., 1967; Pavenstedt, 1967; Sharlin and Shamai, 1990), and most of them also conclude that poverty alone does not cause malfunctioning and extreme distress. Rather, it is the combination of poverty and disorganization that creates what we refer to as families in extreme distress. Pavenstedt (1967) claimed that the only stable pattern in such families is uncertainty. When analyzing the social workers' reports, disorganization in families was coupled with such extreme disorganization in reporting that understanding the data became a difficult task. While telling the story of the families, the social workers tended to jump from one topic to another without completing any one subject. There was confusion of facts with interpretations and evaluations. Sometimes the judgmental attitudes of the workers were introduced as facts, and many details—some of them vital—were left out, as became clear through cross-validating questions asked of social workers and families. Here, for example, is an excerpt from the beginning of a report by H., an experienced social worker:

> I am telling about a family with nine members; two parents and seven children. The oldest son, Sinai, is the mother's son from a previous marriage. The father, Dave, is forty-four years old and unemployed. His wife, Sinai's mother, Ruth, is thirty-three years old and a housekeeper. David and Ruth's remaining children were born in 1975, 1976, 1978, and 1985 [two children were left out]. The father, Dave, was born in Iraq and immigrated to Israel in 1952. The mother, Ruth, was previously married. Six months after Sinai was born, she divorced her husband. Sinai was raised by his grandmother, Ruth's mother, from the age of six months. Now he is living with his mother's family. He served in the army for a year and then got an early

> discharge from military service, using the pretext of personal reasons, his desire to help his mother. . . . All of it is hogwash. He is not a serious person.

The family disorganization was joined and reflected in the social worker's report. Much family data were either missing or incorrect and were presented in an unsystematic manner. The worker began by describing the oldest child, then continued with the father and mother and went back to describe the other children. The question is whether this was due to disorganized data collection owing to the family's condition, or whether it was due to the social worker's belief that the details of the family story were unimportant, since knowing them could not change the situation. Thus, H. did not know whether Dave, the father, had served in the army—a very significant and vital detail in Israeli society. H. assumed that the father had not done military service, an assumption later found to be wrong. Not only had Dave served in the army, but he actually had a good service record.

The faulty assumption made by the worker is a classic example of the halo effect. H. perceived the client as a person who has difficulties in functioning, and he generalized this to include all areas of the client's life. From a therapeutic point of view, Dave's having been able to function for more than two years within a hierarchical and structured environment such as the army, in which pressure and stress are routine, furnishes evidence of the client's strength and should have been used as a source of hope. H. appears not even to have looked for this detail. Even worse, his negative assumption about Dave's army service reveals the generally hopeless attitude H. held about his client.

Similarly, most of the reports by social workers were found either to be missing information or to contain misinformation. Likewise, the professional dealings of the social workers with these clients were marked by a surprising degree of disorganization. Under conditions of disorganization, most activities are impulse determined. This is something we expect to encounter in the behavior of families in extreme distress, but to observe the same pattern in the functioning of the social workers was unexpected. Through narratives, we learn and understand the stress under which the worker operates. It is possible that the feelings of stress expressed in a disorganized worker's narrative can help us understand the deepest human emotions, just as with metaphoric poetry (Eron and Lund, 1993; Sharlin and Shenhar-Alroy, 1987; Sprenkle and Piercy, 1992; Zimmerman and Dickerson, 1994).

This pattern of disorganization is typically observed when working with families in their homes. Members of the family come and go at will. Neighbors come in and are invited to stay even though the family is engaged in discussing intimate and private matters. On the other hand, families invited to the Department of Social Services are unable to commit themselves to a specific date and time.

In similar fashion, a pattern of disorganization and lack of boundaries was observed in many of the Department of Social Services' activities. One example is that of a staff meeting during which H. presented the story of Dave's family. The meeting had been planned three weeks in advance. On the day of the meeting, a number of workers failed to show up because of other activities that suddenly seemed to be more urgent, while others failed to arrive on time. During the meeting, every staff member left the room at some point, each having something else to do: a telephone call, a letter, a short consultation with a secretary or a client. To an outside observer, this might seem identical to the behavior of some clients. Although a contextual view might find a reasonable explanation in job overload and in conflicting scheduling demands commonly experienced in these settings, one cannot overlook the way such behavior would be interpreted by clients.

When trying to understand the factor of disorganization, which affects the coalition of despair, it is important to recognize how it is being imposed on social workers and other mental health professionals by the national policy. From the systemic point of view, professionals are caught between two different systems, namely that of the client and that of the organization. Many social workers and other mental health professionals employed in public service positions are overburdened and often do not have enough organizational support. Being constantly overloaded with many cases that need immediate and urgent solutions does not allow time for careful planning and organization of complicated interventions, such as those needed for families in extreme distress. It is lack of time and resources that often impede peer consultations or adequate supervision. This creates feelings of isolation and causes lack of collaboration among professionals, reducing the sorely needed creativity for working with these families. The common factor of disorganization shared by professionals and families in extreme distress is one aspect of the coalition of despair that affects the ability of the workers to plan and implement an appropriate program of intervention for the clients.

Thinking and Language Patterns

The pattern of interaction found among the families in the project consists of verbal inaccessibility rather than verbal accessibility (Polansky, 1971; Wells, 1981). The serious difficulties in school performance, commonly observed among poor children, are correlated with atypical development of verbal and conceptual skills (Bernstein, 1964).

In reviewing the reports, it was found that the language used by the social workers in describing the families was negative and included many slang words. This was true when workers articulated and explained their own thoughts about the families, as is evident in H.'s story, even though social workers normally use correct and even rich language when expressing themselves on other subjects. It appears that the use of poor language when discussing a family in extreme distress may be another manifestation of the coalition of despair. Shared language is known to be a way of achieving a bond with clients and of entering the culture of a family (Minuchin and Fishman, 1981). However, imitation is not what is meant by the principle of "be where the client is." Some social workers adopt their clients' language and way of thinking without being aware that they are doing it. This seems to have little, if any, function in psychosocial intervention, and it may even prevent the establishment of a professional relationship with the family.

Studies about thinking and cognition indicate that families in extreme distress exhibit poor problem-solving skills (Dohrenwend and Dohrenwend, 1981). Deutch (1963) has argued that these families hardly ever make use of imagination in problem solving and that their way of thinking tends to be simplistic and concrete. Analysis of social workers' reports about their FED clients revealed a similar pattern: their reports are also simplistic and concrete. There is typically a "bad guy," usually the father/husband, who is described as irresponsible, violent, and tyrannical. In most of the reports, the "good guy" is the mother/wife, who is described as being unhappy and suffering because of her husband. This dichotomized picture, shared by the social workers and their clients, represents an unrealistic view. Perceiving the family in such simplistic and concrete terms results in prejudice, with the attendant halo effect, and generalizations that may lead to the desperation and inertia experienced by many of the social workers assigned to such clients. These perceptions have the effect of intensifying conflicts among family members—between the "good" and the "bad" guys of the family story—and preventing the use of imagination and creativity in problem-solving processes (Sharlin and Shamai, 1995).

Absence of creativity in problem solving may well be one of the reasons for the lack of success in working with families in extreme distress. When social workers and mental health professionals lose their creativity and imaginative capabilities in treatment, they join in the clients' way of thinking and become unable to guide their clients or to influence the clients' motivation to function more effectively.

Frustration and Aggression

Frustration among families in extreme distress is primarily expressed through violence. All the reports analyzed included at least one description of a violent episode, either between the couple or toward the children. Most cases had more than one violent episode. Dave, for example, was in jail for two months after he severely battered his wife. Our observations revealed that the wives tended to be verbally violent with their husbands and used both verbal and physical violence with their children. The men expressed their frustration and anger primarily through physical violence.

Social workers, for their part, expressed their anger and frustration in their efforts to deal with these families by using harsh language or labels. Content analysis of social workers' reports revealed the use of cynical turns of phrase in describing the families. For example, H. described Dave, whose body was covered with tattoos, as "a walking art gallery." J., another social worker, wrote that "Mr. A. is suicidal and he is going to have such a sweet death." Later J. explained that A. was diabetic and enjoyed eating chocolate. These remarks were greeted by staff members' laughter. Such comments may be taken as humorous and not necessarily expressions of hostility, but, similar to gallows humor, they can, in fact, serve as adaptive, coping mechanisms by allowing the worker to let off steam in dealing with frustration and despair. However, such expressions or descriptions should be treated by the staff in a responsible and respectful manner.

When presenting their reports, social workers often tended to make negative comments about their clients in the presence of colleagues. We should point out that client families are known to everyone working in the social services agencies involved and that the coalition of despair is reinforced by mutual support between co-workers. It is evident that both social workers and the families they serve are frustrated by their inability to bring about change. Social workers, similar to their clients, expressed their frustration by using abusive language in regard to family members.

Hopelessness and Helplessness

Hopelessness and helplessness are two characteristic features of the client population in our project (Bernstein, Jeremy, and Marcus, 1986; Lewis, 1959, 1961; Pavenstedt, 1965; Polansky et al., 1970; Polansky, 1971; Polansky, Borgman, and De Saix, 1972; Polansky, DeSaix, and Sharlin, 1972; Rosenfeld, 1989). Both also portray social workers' attitudes toward their ability for effective intervention with families in extreme distress. This can be observed in the attitude and behavior of social workers. As noted earlier, missing or inaccurate information was typical of the reports. Negative attitudes were apparent in the workers' conviction that more or less information would make no difference in bringing about change in their clients' lives.

The low self-esteem that characterizes families in extreme distress (Deutch, 1963) is paralleled by some social workers' discrediting their clients. The common ground between the clients' low self-esteem and the negative professional perception of the social workers serves to defeat hope and motivation, both essential ingredients for change. Some social workers found it hard to create a different family story that would include elements of hope, thus becoming a party in maintaining their clients' low self-esteem, despair, hopelessness, and helplessness. Social workers, similar to other helping professionals who provide public services in poor neighborhoods, often feel undervalued. Low salaries and the absence of appropriate supervision, on the one hand, and unwarranted criticism when failing to implement unrealistic tasks, on the other, generate feelings of low self-esteem, often expressed in hopelessness and helplessness. These feelings are conducive to an increasing number of burnout cases among workers. Some eventually leave the profession, whereas many remain but function at a very low level (Friesen and Sarros, 1981; Maslach and Pines, 1977).

An example of hopelessness and helplessness in the behavior of the social workers and their clients is the case of the Ven family and of A., their social worker. A. invited us for a consultation with Mr. Ven, who is an alcoholic. He underwent open-heart surgery nine months before the project began. At the time of the first meeting, Mr. Ven seemed to have given up on life. He rejected any effort toward a helping relationship. As the meetings proceeded, he was offered help at whatever time he might decide he wanted it. He was given the telephone number of the consultant (with the social worker's permission), along with an invitation to call whenever he wished, day or night. Mr. Ven never called for help despite the fact that there was no improvement in his functioning. Meanwhile, A., the social worker, requested a future consultation regarding this family because she found consultations meaningful and helpful for both the family and herself. As with Mr. Ven, she was given the telephone number of one of the consultants, along with permission to call whenever she needed help in working with the family. Although there was no clear improvement in A.'s work with the family, she, similar to her client, never called to ask for help. This may be seen as a case of coalition of despair between the social worker and a family in extreme distress.

The phenomenon of coalition of despair is familiar to people from the mental health professions who work with this population, even if they do not use this term. Professional involvement with the families raises issues related to professional insecurity, thereby arousing fear and a tendency to avoid the involvement altogether. Therefore, purely academic answers to questions about the reasons for not working with these families, as logical and professional as they may be, were not accepted, since they then became a source of more questions and excuses for avoiding the sorely needed professional involvement.

Other issues that need to be addressed in overcoming the fear of professional involvement with distressed families include the personal meaning of meeting with distressed families, the constant awareness of one's professional limitations, and feelings of ineffectiveness and inability to create change. All these doubts leave the social worker, or any other professional, in a state of isolation. It is often very difficult to reveal professional deficiencies and the resultant feelings that are generated. Since only a few social workers and mental health professionals have the necessary fortitude to work with these families, their excuses for hesitating to become involved will focus on the families' resistance and unwillingness to cooperate. These conflicts only increase the families' feelings of loneliness and helplessness. If this is the case, why bother working with this population?

The following section describes a particular therapeutic structure helpful in working with FED.

OVERCOMING THE COALITION OF DESPAIR

Our experience has taught us that it is possible to overcome the coalition of despair and, thereby, the fear of working with families in extreme distress. This can be accomplished by recognizing that working with this population requires a special structuring of the therapeutic agency. This structure has to take into account the complexity of the families as well as the special character of the therapist-client relationship. It calls for (1) special preparation of the therapists before they start working with the families, (2) a model of team intervention, and (3) ongoing supervision, focusing on containing the workers.

Special Preparation of Therapists Before Starting to Work with Families

This special preparation is aimed at changing some of the workers' basic perceptions, which are the source of fear and the coalition of despair, even before intervention begins. Based on past experience, we find that employing narrative perspectives and techniques can be useful in changing the hopelessness and helplessness of the therapists (White, 1990; White and Epston, 1989; Holland, 1991; Borden, 1992; O'Hanlon, 1991). In the first phase of this process, the worker is asked to tell the story of the family, which, as he or she tells it, exposes the meanings and values present in the interaction between the worker and the family. While telling the story, the worker organizes the facts and interpretations into a gestalt that clarifies his or her perception of the family. It is important to let the worker complete the report without any interference, to understand the worker's cognitive and emotional position toward the family (Holland, 1991; Borden, 1992). After completing the story, the worker is asked to indicate the strengths and positive elements he or she has found in the description of the clients. This request provides a basis for changing a negative and hopeless perception into a more positive mode of thinking, one that contains some elements of hope (de Shazer, 1985). Professionals generally find this to be a very difficult task (Sharlin and Shamai, 1990; Shamai and Sharlin, 1996). The task becomes even more difficult when colleagues in the department (acquainted with the families) mention additional negative details about the client, while the worker is trying to focus on strengths. It is therefore important to reinforce positive thinking and to forestall a process that is known as "more of the same" (Watzlawick, Weakland, and Fisch, 1974), that is to say, focusing on weaknesses, pathology, and frustration. After completing the story, the supervisor should provide a summary that emphasizes the family's strengths. Sometimes it is useful to reframe the data to create an option for developing a hopeful attitude (Minuchin and Fishman, 1981). For example, when the social worker described Dave's family, he mentioned that Dave asked him to persuade Ruth, the wife, not to send the children to a religious boarding school because they were not religious and it would be better for the children to be raised at home. In the summary of H.'s story, Dave's request was stressed because it revealed a lot of caring on the part of the husband for his children. Focusing on this issue led to some positive thinking among the social workers, who concluded that Dave wanted to keep the family together, as otherwise he would not have sought H.'s help.

In the second phase, a new dialogue with the family is created. The meeting with the family at this phase is led by the supervisor, while the other member of the professional team acts as a participant observer who focuses on hopeful elements that are brought up in the session. The supervisor encourages the family to focus on strengths rather than on pathology to show that hope is possible. Using elements from the de Shazer approach is very helpful at this stage (de Shazer, 1985). For example, A., the Ven family's social worker, told the supervisor after the session that she used to get very angry at Mr. Ven's egocentric lifestyle and irresponsible behavior toward his family, but during the family's interview with the supervisor, she realized how deeply depressed Mr. Ven was and began to feel compassion for him. She now understood that what he needed was a great deal of help rather than criticism. Moreover, the simplistic view she had of the family changed as well. The social worker also realized that Mrs. Ven was not always the "good guy"—it was very easy to see how she deprived her husband of any authority.

In the third phase, the family worker is asked to tell the story of the family once again, as if the story had not been heard before, and differences in the structure and language of the narrative are elaborated. This is done to focus on areas that might lead to a constructive dialogue between the worker and the family. Another technique that is helpful in this phase is the use of metaphors. The worker is asked to offer a metaphor for the therapeutic system as he or she perceives it, before and after the session with the supervisor. The changes in the metaphor should be analyzed, as well as the reasons that are behind the changes. For example, O. saw the family as a kindergarten group and herself as a teacher who is expected to relate to and love all the children (family members) alike. However, she felt she could not live up to this expectation, as she resented a specific family member (the father). According to O., the father demanded a lot but was not ready to make an effort. The supervisor did not change the kindergarten metaphor but enabled O. to find something positive about her attitude toward the father. She became aware of the resentment and wanted to find its function in the therapeutic system. This allowed her to continue her intervention with the family.

At times, social workers are too quick to change their metaphors or stories from ones of helplessness to ones of hope. When this happens, it is important to point the way back to reality. Such occurrences usually indicate that many "hopeless" variables are present in working with families in extreme distress. An extreme reversal of attitude is a continuation of the coalition process, since the worker's thinking about the family remains concrete and simplistic. Overcoming the coalition of despair does not mean ignoring the complex and difficult challenges faced in working with these clients.

A Model of Team Intervention

Team intervention allows for some division of the overwhelming tasks involved in working with families in extreme distress. Teamwork creates the conditions that prevent workers' feelings of isolation. It facilitates the sharing of feelings such as disappointment, hopelessness, and helplessness with other members, thus protecting workers from feeling isolated when working with families in extreme distress. It is further assumed that personal and professional differences among team members would prevent the formation of multiple coalitions of despair, thus enabling mutual support among team members. Also, teamwork provides opportunities for brainstorming among workers to find ways to avoid an impasse in the intervention process.

Ongoing Supervision and Support of the Workers

It is important to assure the worker that ongoing supervision or consultations will be available. This may reduce the fear of isolation workers experience when working with distressed families. One important dimension of supervision is sustaining the therapeutic team.* The overwhelming situations that characterize families in extreme distress are expressed in the content and process of the intervention. Often, the team has to relate to unexpected crises which consume the family's energy and which do not leave room for continuing the planned therapeutic procedure.

Let us illustrate through the case of the S. family. The therapeutic contract focused on strengthening the parents' marital communication skills and finding some arrangement to help with their financial debts. To the social worker, it appeared that intervention would help resolve the financial issue and that the couple could concentrate on developing constructive communication between them. Unfortunately, the plan was disrupted when the family found out that the judge was not ready to accept the proposed arrangement for paying their debts, which meant Mr. S.'s possible arrest, just when his three-year-old daughter had to undergo an unexpected operation. Mr. and Mrs. S. were afraid and did not know how to prepare the little girl for her operation, and neither did they have the energy to go through with it.

When relating to one case, such a crisis can be contained by one person, but when such crises become the norm, they exhaust the social worker. Also, such norms might become an obstacle to working on a deeper level, for example, when trying to help build the family's coping resilience. All of this might erode the therapist's and the team's faith in their ability to help the family and lessen their professional self-esteem. It is the role of the supervisor, then, to contain the team's disappointment, anger, and despair, thus preventing such feelings from ruling the relationship with the family and creating a coalition of despair.

One of the basic elements in working with families in extreme distress is overcoming the fear and the coalition of despair that the social worker and the therapist connect with experiences of failure and isolation and changing them into a *coalition of hope*. It is therefore necessary to be in touch with the fear, anger, and sometimes even rejection of this population. It is further important to check out issues of countertransference and intersubjectivity that

*There are many dimensions to supervision, which will be described and discussed in Chapter 9.

arise in meetings between families in distress and the therapist. Such self-examination by the therapist and the team can help sharpen their understanding of the family's world of experiences and feelings, thereby reducing anger and rejection and facilitating the creation of a therapeutic dialogue toward hope.

DEVELOPING A MODEL FOR WORKING WITH FED

Based on acquired know-how in intervention with FED, it seems that certain principles are crucial for effective intervention. These are (1) team intervention, (2) a focused and structured therapeutic process with a clear goal and of limited time, and (3) therapeutic sessions conducted at the family's home to reduce the family's absenteeism.

Team Intervention

As mentioned earlier in this chapter, intervention with FED can be overwhelming, often requiring the therapist to play many implementation roles. Usually, just one person, who might easily enter into a coalition of despair, cannot accomplish this. Therefore, teamwork is recommended. There are different ways of creating teams. We recommend that the team include two professionals. One professional should take the role of case manager and be responsible for providing the family with the necessary aid, establishing a support system, and linking the family with community institutions that are relevant to the family's functioning. (Generally, case managers are either on staff at a social services department or affiliated with one.) The second professional should assume the role of family therapist and also be the team leader in charge of conducting the therapeutic meetings with the family. It is necessary for both members of the team to be present at the therapeutic meetings, for two reasons: one, they can become a model for direct and respectful communication, and, two, they can insist on clear boundaries regarding the issues that the family brings to the session. Financial issues, for example, are dealt with mostly by the case manager, whereas issues concerning the relationship among family members are handled by the family therapist. Such clear boundaries in role description help create an organized context, which could also influence the family's organization.

Applying Team Intervention in a Mental Health Clinic

In this situation, it would be helpful to have contact with the social worker assigned to the family and to ask him or her to organize an intervention team. Sometimes this works, but in most cases, lack of funds or some political excuse will stand in the way. Consequently, it would help to establish whatever contact is possible with the family's social worker, divide the tasks and roles, and present them to the family. It is important to maintain open communication between the two professionals, to prevent isolation of either one. If creating a team is not possible, it might be helpful to use intensive supervision, including life supervision, or to collaborate with a colleague involved in the process, to prevent isolation and the formation of a coalition of despair.

Focused and Structured Therapeutic Process with a Clear Goal and of Limited Time

Since disorganization is one of FED's basic characteristics, it is helpful to create a structured and clear therapeutic context, with a well-defined goal and a predetermined time frame. Because of the severity and complexity of the problems presented by FED, which often require long periods of intervention, establishing a series of short interventions is suggested. This would include ten meetings of intensive intervention (about three per month), followed by a three-month period of maintenance and another intensive period, if necessary.

Conduct the Therapeutic Sessions at the Family's Home

It is important to remember that not showing up for meetings does not mean the family is unmotivated. Absenteeism is often due to family members' general disorganization and lack of effective time-organizing skills. Therefore, meeting the family at home helps avoid this problem, and also reveals important therapeutic information because the process takes place in the family's natural environment. Another reason for conducting therapeutic sessions in the family's home is to alleviate any suspicions about helping professionals that the family may have accumulated from painful and ineffective past experiences. Thus, conducting the sessions "on the family's turf" gives the family the status of host and reduces the hierarchical gap between the family and the therapeutic team. It is important for the therapist to understand that missed therapeutic sessions are mostly a result of disorganization rather than resistance to therapy or lack of motivation. If the family prefers meeting at the clinic, the sessions are, of course, conducted there.

PART III: ASSESSMENT OF FED

Chapter 4

Descriptive Scale of Families in Extreme Distress

As mentioned in the literature review, many attempts have been made to measure and specifically assess poor, disorganized families. The difficulty of assessing such families has no doubt been a major obstacle to conducting a clinical inquiry in the area. Generalizations about disorganized families or multiproblem families have led to many misconceptions. A descriptive scale may contribute to overcoming some of these difficulties.

We prefer to call these families FED, since, in our minds, they represent much more than a multiplicity of problems or disorganization. We use the definition of families in extreme distress because it is a complex concept, involving more than either of the other terms, multiproblem families or disorganized families. The label FED includes the presence of multiple problems and disorganization, as well as the interaction effects of these problems.

From the literature review, we found that there is no clear definition of FED that is universally accepted. Dax and Hagger (1977) claimed that even though many definitions have been applied to multiproblem families, the very fact that these families have so many problems does not allow a precise definition, but only a general characterization. It is, therefore, far better to describe their characteristics, so that when reviewing the various descriptions accorded to these families, we find major factors common to them all. They live from day to day and usually in poverty, since they are unable to manage their lives. Their debts are high, incurred through expenses for housekeeping, shopping, rent, and often gambling.

Usually, these are large families that are always on the move. Family members work in temporary jobs or whenever jobs are available, generally in part-time positions. They are usually unskilled and remain unemployed most of the time. Their homes are often unkempt and neglected and do not meet hygienic standards. Proper household management does not exist, and meals are never on time. Violence in the family and quarrels between the spouses, often drug abusers, typically take place in front of the children. Dependence on social services is chronic.

We wanted to find out whether this description of FED is still valid when referring to this population in the 1990s. The need to revalidate past descriptions was reinforced by a family therapist who took part in the project. She claimed that two of the families assigned to the program should not be defined as multiproblem families, but rather as families with severe problems that affect certain aspects of their functioning. Following Dax and Hagger (1977), we attempted to delineate a specific description of families defined as multiproblem families, disorganized families, and families in extreme distress (see Figure 4.1).

FROM FED DESCRIPTION TO FED SCALE: A CLINICAL ASSESSMENT

With the intention of deriving a specific description of FED, we asked for a list of the problems faced by each family in the program. From these lists, we gleaned nine problem areas (categories) that most characterized FED: poverty, housing, health, couple functioning, parental functioning, children, substance abuse, antisocial behavior, and support systems. Each category included between four and eight items describing the specific problems involved in the category. This was the basis for developing a descriptive scale for assessing families in extreme distress. FED are characterized by at least five out of the nine criteria, or by at least twenty-two issues marked in all nine categories (Sharlin and Shamai, 1990). It was interesting to note that the two families assessed by the family

FIGURE 4.1. FED Categories and Criteria

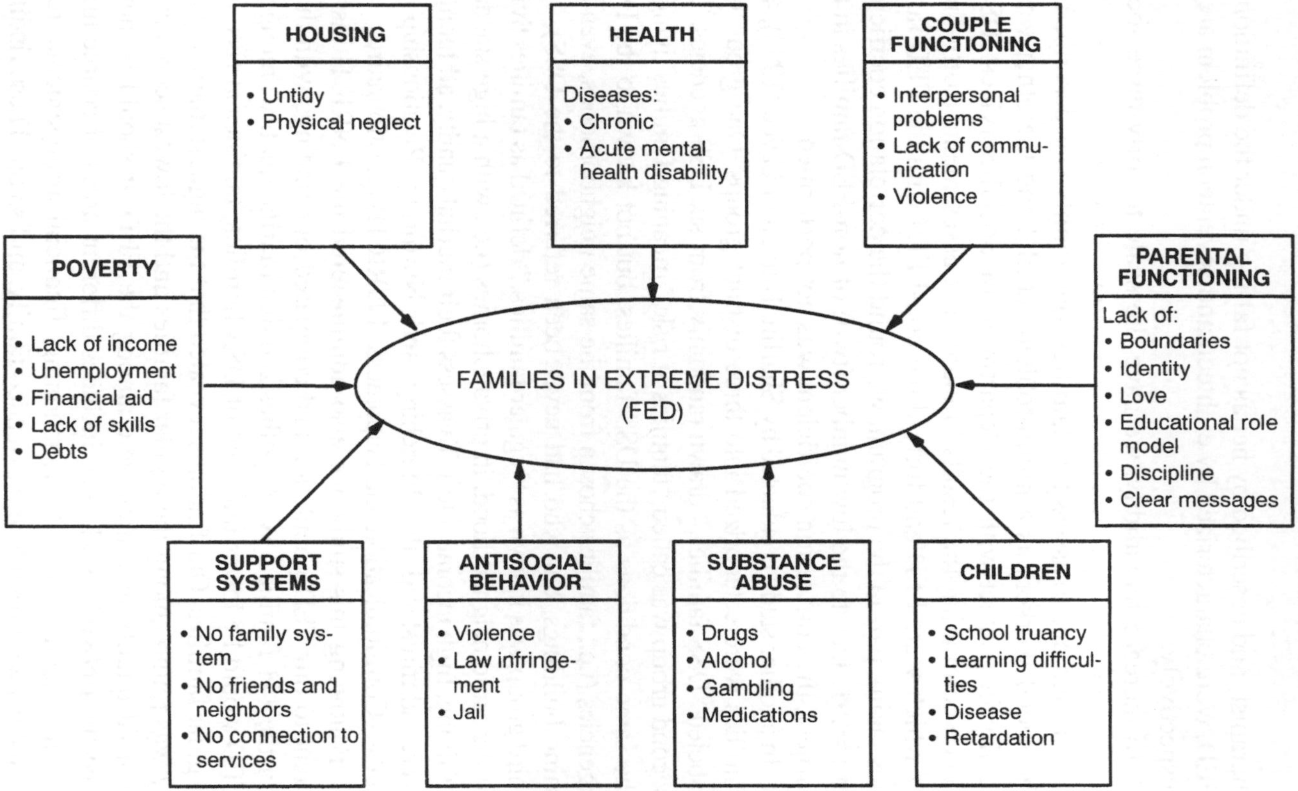
HOUSING
• Untidy
• Physical neglect
HEALTH
Diseases:
• Chronic
• Acute mental health disability
COUPLE FUNCTIONING
• Interpersonal problems
• Lack of communication
• Violence
POVERTY
• Lack of income
• Unemployment
• Financial aid
• Lack of skills
• Debts
FAMILIES IN EXTREME DISTRESS (FED)
PARENTAL FUNCTIONING
Lack of:
• Boundaries
• Identity
• Love
• Educational role model
• Discipline
• Clear messages
SUPPORT SYSTEMS
• No family system
• No friends and neighbors
• No connection to services
ANTISOCIAL BEHAVIOR
• Violence
• Law infringement
• Jail
SUBSTANCE ABUSE
• Drugs
• Alcohol
• Gambling
• Medications
CHILDREN
• School truancy
• Learning difficulties
• Disease
• Retardation

therapist, and described by her as not falling under the definition of FED, were characterized by eighteen and seventeen problem areas, respectively.

To increase its validity, we gave the scale to forty-three social workers and family therapists from various clinics and services. We asked each one to assess two families: one family was described by the social workers as a multiproblem family, and the other was a family in contact with the Department of Social Services (DSS). When comparing the results of eighty-six assessments (forty-three of which were FED and forty-three non-FED) with the FED families taking part in the program, we found the correlation coefficient of $r = .91$. Due to the low number (two) of non-FED families in the project, the correlation coefficient was not performed.

In another study conducted by Sharlin, Katz, and Lavee (1992), 441 families were categorized into three distinct groups. One group was labeled "DSS families," drawn randomly from six DSS agencies. The second group was called "families at risk," meaning families living in the same conditions as the DSS families, but not known to the DSS agencies (i.e., families chosen from the same neighborhoods, even the same buildings, but who had never been referred to the DSS). The third group was known as "regular families," defined as families living in the same neighborhood, in private homes (i.e., with a high standard of living, high income, etc.). To assess their marital quality, all families were administered the Enriching and Nurturing Relationship Issues—Communication and Happiness (ENRICH) questionnaire.

Following this study, we also administered the ENRICH instrument to our FED population and compared our findings with those for the 441 families. We hypothesized that marital quality among the FED would be lower than that of DSS families, families at risk, and regular families. Our findings revealed that the highest marital quality was found among the regular families and the lowest scores in all marital quality measures were among the FED. It should be noted that the ENRICH scale also includes different areas of couple functioning, such as parental functioning, financial arrangements, relationships with friends and extended family, and so on. These findings may provide construct validity for our FED descriptive scale.

THE FAMILIES IN EXTREME DISTRESS SCALE

The Families in Extreme Distress Scale is a simple additive scale that can be easily used by a social worker who knows the family. When this is not the case, and the family is unknown, each test area can be included in a structured interview for completion of the scale.

As noted earlier, the scale has nine categories. Each category includes several items, all presented negatively, as they may apply to the family under study. If an item does describe the situation in the family, then the number 1 should be entered. If this item is nonexistent in the family, then 0 should be entered. For instance, poverty, the first category, has eight items. The scoring range for this test area is from 0—meaning no such item in this family—to 8—meaning that all indicated items exist in this family. As a rule, each category with three or more items is considered an FED category for the family under study, unless otherwise indicated; for example, the categories of substance abuse and health (see Figure 4.2). Each qualifying category should be marked with an X next to the category name. A total of all items marked on the scale should be calculated. To meet the definition of FED, the family must be characterized by at least five out of the nine categories presented in Figure 4.2, or by at least twenty-two items marked in all nine categories.

The FED scale may serve several additional purposes. First, it allows us to assess whether this is indeed an FED case, and then to apply the clinical interventions described in this book. Another possible use is a functional evaluation of the family to obtain a general picture of where the family stands and what the focus of the intervention should be. Finally, the scale may serve as an evaluative instrument for learning what has been achieved, what improvements have been made, how the treatment has progressed, and what else should be done. Our ability to be more precise in evaluating such families may also protect clinicians from becoming overwhelmed by the families' problems. Inasmuch as we lump these families in a category—FED—we should bear in mind that families in extreme distress may differ from one another. Follow-up should be done with each individual family assessed on the FED scale so that changes and/or progress can be observed.

FIGURE 4.2. The Families in Extreme Distress Scale

1. **Poverty (   )**

a. No income from work	______
b. Unemployed	______
c. No professional training	______
d. Work when available	______
e. Income maintenance	______
f. Debts	______
g. Impaired family budget	______
h. Lacking basic supplies	______
Total score for poverty	______

Note: To count this test area, at least three items should be checked. If the total score is higher than 3, then mark the name of the test area with an X.

2. **Housing (   )**

a. Home in disarray	______
b. Physical neglect (bad smell, dirty walls)	______
c. No heat in the winter	______
d. Condensed living quarters	______
e. At least one of the following utilities is disconnected: water/electricity/gas/telephone	______
f. House caught fire	______
Total score for housing	______

Note: To count this test area, at least three items should be checked.

3. **Health (   )**

a. Acute illness—every week or two	______
b. Chronic illness	______
c. Mental illness	______
d. Disability (physical or mental)	______
e. Depression	______
f. Psychiatric hospitalization	______

g. Attempted suicide _______

h. Terminal illness _______

Total score for health ________

Note: One item is enough to count this area.

4. Couple Functioning (   )

a. Marital relationship problems _______

b. Extramarital affairs _______

c. Lack of communication _______

d. Physical violence toward spouse _______

e. Verbal violence _______

f. Problems in sexual relations _______

g. Absence of role differentiation _______

Total score for couple functioning ________

Note: To count this test area, at least three items should be checked.

5. Parental Functioning (   )

a. Absence of boundaries _______

b. No parental figure for a role model _______

c. No educational figure _______

d. Conditional love _______

e. Impaired discipline _______

f. Lack of clear messages _______

g. Violence toward children _______

h. Suspicion of incest _______

Total score for parental functioning ________

Note: To count this area, at least three items should be checked.

6. Children (   )

a. Multiple-children families _______

b. Truancy from educational institutions _______

c. Learning difficulties _______

FIGURE 4.2 (*continued*)

d. Running away from school _______
e. Illness _______
f. Retardation _______
g. Disability _______
h. Delinquency _______
i. Behavioral difficulties _______
j. Sibling violence _______
k. Parental physical abuse _______
l. Physical and/or emotional child neglect _______

Total score for children _______

Note: To count this area, at least three items should be checked.

7. Substance Abuse ( )

a. Drugs _______
b. Alcohol _______
c. Gambling _______
d. Medication abuse _______

Total score for substance abuse _______

Note: One item is enough to count this area.

8. Antisocial Behavior ( )

a. Under arrest _______
b. In prison _______
c. Lack of communication _______
d. Violence against social institutions _______
e. Violating the law _______
f. Awaiting trial _______
g. Running away from home _______

Total score for antisocial behavior _______

Note: To count this area, at least three items should be checked.

9. Support Systems (   )

a. No support from extended family _______

b. No support from friends and neighbors _______

c. No relationship with the Department of Social Services _______

d. No relationship with other institutions in the community _______

Total score for support systems _______

Note: To count this area, at least three items should be checked.

Total number of items _______

Total number of categories _______

PART IV: INTERVENTION TECHNIQUES

Chapter 5

Developing a Toolbox and Creating the Therapeutic Context

The word toolbox may invoke many images. Some people might imagine a handyman who uses tools to fix some technical problem. Taken in this context, it suggests neither emotional involvement nor a humanistic attitude, both of which are significant components of therapy. Others may relate to this image as a useful box, the contents of which—the tools—have been collected over the years and are used by the owner with caring and joy. Our notion of a toolbox relates to the means used by therapists to implement creative interventions. Not only do therapists use these tools with joy and pleasure, but they develop different ways of activating the tools and, in so doing, create "multiform and multitask tools." Furthermore, since various combinations can be created simultaneously using different tools, there is an ongoing opportunity for changing and enriching the quality of the tools and their use. Those therapists who perceive the toolbox as a means of enabling and creating are excited to acquire new tools, to expand their repertoire, and to discover as many ways of operating the tools as possible. However, they are also aware of a very basic fact: behind each tool is a person who creates and operates it. It is the human mind, consisting of cognitive and emotional domains, that affects and determines the way in which the tool will be activated and used. Therefore, when relating to the toolbox in this way, it becomes not only a source of technical skills but also a combination of cognitive, emotional, and behavioral systems that are used in the process of creating and implementing therapeutic interventions.

Pinkston and associates (1982) define techniques as "means for change agents to carry out a procedure through intervention steps"

(p. 52). This definition is a good example of the complexity involved in defining the term technique within the context of therapy in general and family therapy in particular. Sometimes it is described in relation to logistical questions, such as the following:

1. Who is invited to the therapeutic session? Some family therapists insist on meeting with the entire family and may even cancel a meeting if one or two members are unable to participate, whereas others may meet the family and discuss the meaning of the absence of specific members
2. Who is conducting the therapy? There may be one family therapist, cotherapist, or an observing team, originally introduced as part of the Milan approach (Boscolo et al., 1987), in which a group is involved in creating an intervention while the therapist serves as "a messenger." Other approaches, such as structural and experiential ones (Minuchin, 1974; Satir and Baldwin, 1983; Whitaker, 1967), focus on the central place of the therapist, who conducts the treatment and defines the different roles of the cotherapists in concrete terms.
3. What is the length of the therapeutic session and the frequency of the therapeutic meetings? Some approaches suggest long periods between meetings, assuming that change takes place at home, whereas others are based on change within the meetings themselves and therefore require weekly sessions with the family.

In other contexts, techniques are connected with theoretical assumptions, that is, whether the change involves action or insight. Approaches that assert change as an action will focus on techniques that call for overt activity within the family, such as enactment, guided communication, structuring, and restructuring (Minuchin and Fishman, 1981). At the other extreme are approaches that focus on reaching an alternative understanding of the problem and its causes, thereby resulting in different kinds of interpretations. Regarding theoretical assumptions about the role of the therapists, are they "neutral," as required by the Milan approach (Boscolo et al., 1987), or are they involved, as with Whitaker (1967) and Minuchin (1974)?

When we refer to technique in the treatment of families in extreme distress, we focus on the following questions: What does the therapy concretely accomplish within the session? What are its implications for the family? Although we differentiate issues of context from technique, both of them have to be taken into consideration when evaluating the therapeutic process. The complexity of FED does not allow our being limited to techniques that are connected to a specific intervention approach; rather, we must take advantage of as many means as possible to challenge the family to change. The terms tool and toolbox emphasize our perception that everything that can work toward change within FED should be used, unless it creates unethical results, such as humiliation of the family, inhibition of personal desires, and so forth. Therefore, we have "collected" many tools which seem to be useful in working with FED and which may provide a secure base for therapists during their uncertain journey with clients from this population. If one perceives the toolbox as a system of humanistic techniques and skills, then it appears dynamic rather than cold and distant.

However, this perception of the toolbox calls for a change in the therapist's way of thinking—it requires modesty. This might be difficult, since members of our professional community often prefer discussions and analyses of cases based on complicated and abstract assumptions and theories. Here, we suggest an alternative direction, something very concrete, based on one simple assumption: if it works, then use it! Furthermore, the complexity of FED does not necessarily require complicated and abstract intervention approaches and techniques, nor can treatment be limited to one intervention approach or one set of techniques. We are talking about the ability to be practical rather than sophisticated, although when working with FED, being practical is sometimes connected with sophisticated thinking.

Therefore, we use different techniques without limiting ourselves to any particular intervention approaches. A variety of techniques aim to increase insight and understanding, whereas many others emphasize actions. Likewise, there are situations in which the therapists are more neutral, although in most cases, we find them to be very actively involved. In some instances, they give direct advice or instructions, whereas in other cases, they take an empowering approach, encouraging the family to find its own strength and creativity. It is the specific character of the family within a given situation that determines the choice of a specific technique in relation to the goal of the session or that of the entire intervention. To implement this approach, it is necessary to have a wide set of techniques or tools at one's disposal.

As Minuchin and Fishman (1981) have suggested, it is difficult to describe one technique as separate from others, since each technique may consist of a combination of different techniques. For example, to create or increase direct communication among family members, the therapist must either model such communication or empower them to find a way to do it, while at the same time supporting, reinforcing, and reflecting their efforts. The process resembles a puzzle in which one piece does not make any sense until it is connected with some other pieces; only then do we get some idea about the entire picture.

PREPARATORY AND GOAL-ORIENTED TECHNIQUES

A qualitative study was carried out to analyze the therapeutic process within the project (Gilad-Smolinsky, 1996). Every session in the project was tape-recorded and underwent a word-by-word transcription; some meetings were also videotaped. The data were intended to identify the therapeutic techniques that were being used. Two main intervention categories were identified. The first category describes tools that aim to create a context within which the family will be able to work toward change: these tools are called "preparing tools." The second category describes tools that aim to create a specific, desired change in the family: these tools are called "goal-oriented tools."

The preparing tools include techniques such as supporting, modeling, and using communication skills as various means for facilitating the initiation and continuation of the therapeutic process. As found by Gilad-Smolinsky (1996), these techniques were used in about two-thirds of the intervention approaches that were implemented throughout the entire therapeutic process. This extended use is explained by the character of the families in extreme distress and by the type of relationships they create within their environment.

The need for these techniques is defined by their disorganization and lack of stability, which often makes it difficult, or even impossible, to continue with the intervention (Minuchin et al., 1967; Rabin, 1989; Rosenthal, 1974; Schlosberg and Kagan, 1988; Wells, 1981). Therefore, it is the role of the therapist to enable continuation of the therapeutic process by any means available. The main characteristic of all preparing techniques is the emotional acceptance of the family, including its negative attitudes and behaviors toward the therapist. The ability of the therapist to interpret rejecting attitudes and behaviors, such as fear, distress, and mistrust that have been accumulated by the family through its experience allows the therapist to be with the family without entering into either a defensive or offensive position, both of which mean distancing from the family. The following case can serve as an illustration.

Case Illustration

The team, which included a family therapist and a case manager, received a phone call from Mrs. A. about an hour before their meeting. Mrs. A. told the team that she and her husband had had a fight and that he would not be at home for the meeting, suggesting that it be canceled. Furthermore, she added that things had not changed and that she did not believe someone could really help them. It was clear from her voice that Mrs. A. was full of anger and despair, and the team reflected to her that they did hear her feelings. They shared with Mrs. A. their own disappointment. They were ready and anxious to meet with the family, especially after the last session, in which it had been clear how much the members of the family cared about one another, in spite of the severe financial stress affecting their existence. The team reminded Mrs. A. that they had a joint contract to find ways to overcome the financial stress, as well as to work on parenting issues so that she and her husband could be a more effective parental team. The team told Mrs. A. that they believed in the family's ability to create a warm and supportive environment for the children and to facilitate the growth and development of the entire family. Mrs. A. responded to this encouragement by saying "From your mouth to God's ears"; thus, it was clear that she had calmed down and was ready to accept the team's positive attitude. The team sensed the change in Mrs. A.

and requested that she find her husband, tell him about the discussion, and convince him to attend the session, even at a later hour. Mrs. A. said she knew where to find him, but did not know how to approach him in such a way that he would listen to her. The family therapist suggested that Mrs. A. ask her husband just to listen to what had transpired in the discussion with the team. She emphasized to Mrs. A. that before inviting him to the session, it might help to tell Mr. A. that she knew he cared about the family and that the financial distress was leaving both of them vulnerable and sometimes with a very "short fuse," readily leading to counterproductive fights. The family therapist expressed her trust in the ability of Mrs. A. to use her suggestion and to modify it according to her deep understanding of her husband. Mrs. A. was ready to try, but was not sure she could succeed.

After about twenty minutes, Mrs. A. called again to say that her husband came back home and would attend the session, even though he did not believe that the Department of Social Services really wanted to help them. Mrs. A. seemed to be angry again and had joined in her husband's attitude in relating to the family therapist and the case manager as representatives of a hated institution. The team heard the anger in Mrs. A.'s words, but they chose to focus on the ability of the family to reorganize in a short time and to accept the challenge of the session.

When the team arrived at the A. house, they were received with offensive behavior on the part of both Mr. and Mrs. A. It seems that they were a target for the anger and despair in which the couple could join together. The previous containment of Mrs. A. through support and modeling enabled the family to come to the session, but was not enough to allow its continuation. There was a need for further preparing techniques before the A.s would be able to focus on the goals they had set for themselves. The team reflected to Mr. and Mrs. A. that they felt the anger and despair in the room and asked them whether they were ready to share and verbalize it.

Mr. A. began by attacking the Department of Social Services for not being willing to help them. After his wife joined in, both of them were so focused on attacking the department that they could not relate to any comments made by the case manager, who was trying to redirect them toward their own problems. At that point, the family therapist began to share with the team, in front of the family, her perception of Mr. and Mrs. A.; they were not only very angry and despairing but also afraid of being disappointed again. Since their history with the department was a painful one, they were obviously wondering whether they could trust the team or whether it was going to be yet another painful experience. Mr. and Mrs. A. agreed with the team about their mistrust and fear of being disappointed again, and the team then reassured them that such feelings were quite normal. The case manager suggested writing an agreement with the team concerning the goals of the intervention, specifying areas in which the Department of Social Services could help prevent another disappointment. Mr. and Mrs. A. thought it might be a good idea.

* * *

In fact, this was a repetition of the therapeutic goals that were stated in the previous session, but the long history of painful experiences with institutions in the community, combined with the disorganized character of the family, required further communication and clarification of these goals. If the team had not allowed this process to happen, by attempting to justify the department's behavior or by responding with an angry attitude toward the family's inability to commit and their tendency to create so many difficulties, the session and the entire therapeutic process would have been rendered ineffective. The unconditional support and acceptance shown by the team allowed the communication to continue and re-created the therapeutic context.

Gilad-Smolinsky (1996) describes the category of preparing techniques as a necessary stage, such as those in the human developmental life cycle. Similar to every individual, these families need, first and foremost, to feel that they are in a safe environment as the basis for experiencing new cognitive, emotional, and behavioral skills. Families in extreme distress are often lacking a solid and safe base; they have instead a painful and unstable one. Therefore, they need to be given an opportunity to create a safe context, and it is the role of the therapist to allow and contain the experience of building it. Since the domain of preparing techniques has a significant effect on enabling the therapeutic process, we view this set of techniques as the core tools for intervention with families in extreme distress. As previously stated, it is not only supporting, not only modeling, and not only using communication skills that make up this toolbox; rather, it includes an entire system of humanistic techniques and skills to be employed in various combinations, as dictated by each individual situation.

The second category is goal-oriented techniques that aim to develop communication skills among family members, to focus on specific tasks, to organize daily routines, and to reframe and relabel situations. These techniques are widely used by family therapists with other types of families as well. With FED, these techniques are generally used during only one-third of the intervention process because the beginning of each therapeutic session is characterized by the use of preparatory tools. The implementation of goal-oriented techniques is possible only after the context is made safe enough for the family.

* * *

In their fifth meeting, Mr. A. received the team with a smile and told them that he had accepted their suggestion and applied for a job in a hotel, located close to their town, where his wife could also find work. Mr. and Mrs. A. saw this opportunity as a good way to overcome their financial stress, especially after the case manager helped them to make a new arrangement for paying back their loan. Nevertheless, Mrs. A. was afraid that taking a job would multiply her responsibilities; she feared that she would have to shoulder the burden of household chores and child care duties by herself after working seven hours at the hotel. The team applauded the couple for finding the jobs and attempting to overcome their financial stress. They reassured Mrs. A. that her fear was a valid one shared by many dual-career families with young children. The family therapist suggested that Mrs. A. verbalize her fear to Mr. A. and that both of them make an effort to create a plan allowing them to take the jobs without giving up their desire to function as a team in rearing the children:

Mr. A.: I don't know what she is talking about. When I did not work, she complained and said she would go to work, and when I found a job for me and for her, she continues to complain.

Mrs. A.: I know what will happen. I will work from 8 a.m. until 3 p.m. Before I go to work, I'll go crazy. I'll wake up the children, help them get dressed, prepare them hot chocolate, take them to kindergarten, and run quickly so I won't miss the bus; then when I finish working, I'll have to run so I won't be late at the kindergarten, take the kids home and be with them, and, at the same time, cook, clean the house, do the laundry and the shopping. You will sleep until 1 p.m. and then you will go to work until 11 p.m. . . .

Mr. A.: So, if you don't want to, then don't take the job.

Family Therapist (FT): What you are doing right now won't help you to solve the problem. It is clear you are somehow disappointed that Mrs. A. was not so happy with your finding her a job, but she raised a problem that exists in many families, including mine, and it can be worked out. Did you hear from Mrs. A. that she rejected your suggestion?

Mr. A.: Well, I don't know . . .

Mrs. A.: No, I did not reject it; I want to go out and take the job, but I want him to help me with the household and with the kids.

Mr. A.: First of all, I will work only every other week in the afternoon. So, when I work in the morning, I can wake up the children and take them to kindergarten while you arrange things in the house. [To the team] For her, the house has to be like a museum; she does not let us breathe . . .

Mrs. A.: If I didn't do it, we would live like animals in the trash.

FT: [Addressing the couple] It seems you are trying to close another issue here, but we are not finished with finding a joint solution to overcome the new situation. You were just in the middle of suggesting a way.

Mr. A.: Yes. So when both of us work in the morning, I can take care of the children in the morning before leaving home, pick them up from kindergarten, and spend time with them.

FT: Yes, you are very creative in playing with them.

Mr. A.: But I don't want you [Mrs. A.] to interrupt us every five minutes to say that there is a mess. When we finish playing, we will clean up and put everything back in place.

Mrs. A.: What will happen when you work in the afternoon?

Mr. A.: This will be a difficult week. However, you have to remember that the children are eating their main meal at kindergarten, and we will eat at the hotel, so you can give them only a light supper and not get crazy about cooking. I agree to get up at 10 a.m. and do the shopping, if you leave me a list, do the laundry, if you prepare it according to the colors, and arrange the house—but my way. But I won't get up at 6 a.m. to help with the children after working until 11 p.m. and going to sleep at midnight.

Mrs. A.: You will do all these things? I doubt it.

FT: [To Mrs. A.] Are you ready to give it a chance?

Mrs. A.: Yes, but I do not believe it.

FT: How do you plan to give Mr. A. a real chance?

Mrs. A.: I don't know. After such a long experience, it's difficult.

FT: Let's try to think together. Did your husband suggest this kind of help sometime in the past, or is this something new?

Mrs. A.: To tell the truth, this is the first time he ever offered to help me, and I hope it will work.

FT: So, you are talking about a new experience for the family. Mr. A. is suggesting that he assume new roles that are related to your goal of creating a parental team and reducing financial stress. How can you [to Mrs. A.] support him in doing this? How would you, Mr. A., want to be supported?

Mr. A.: I want her to tell me sometimes that I am doing things right and not always to criticize me. Can you do it?

Mrs. A.: [Smiles]

Mr. A.: [Laughs] Well, this might be more difficult for her than doing everything by herself.

Mrs. A.: You may be surprised.

FT: It seems to me that you have succeeded in working out a good plan, let's see how it will work and where you will have to make changes—but this was a wonderful display of teamwork by both of you.

As illustrated, the team could work with the A.s toward a specific goal only after the family felt safe within the therapeutic context. This safety was achieved through intensive containment during the previous four meetings, as well as by advocacy-type intervention on the part of the case manager, who helped Mr. A. to rearrange the conditions of their loan repayment and to find employment. The integration of these two aspects turned the therapeutic context into a challenging process rather than a threatening one, thereby encouraging communication between Mr. and Mrs. A. that focused on problem-solving activity.

In regard to the specific tools, we can also divide them into tools that affect the entire therapeutic context and those which effect change. The tools that help to create the therapeutic context are joining, structuring, and creating boundaries. Although these tools are also used to effect change, other tools available for use in creating change include empowering, suggestive techniques, framing and reframing of family myths and narratives, modeling, and enhancing communication skills. None of these techniques are new in either psychotherapy or family therapy, but their implementation with families in extreme distress calls for special attention. Let us illustrate the use of some of these tools.

PREPARATORY TECHNIQUES

Joining

Minuchin and Fishman (1981) describe joining as a process by which the therapist joins the family in an attempt to learn the family language and experience from inside, even though this language and experience are different from his or her own life experience. When relating to families in extreme distress, joining means being able to feel and understand the meaning of uncertainty, disorganization, and lack of stability, without becoming overwhelmed by it. Moreover, it means using this understanding as a tool for leading the family in overcoming its distress.

Case Illustration

During the first meeting with the B. family, the team brought a video camera, since the family had agreed to allow the session to be taped. As Mrs. B. saw the team approaching, she began to yell at them for bringing the camera; Mr. B. joined her, as did Mrs. B.'s sister, who had come to visit them. The young children began to cry, and Mrs. B.'s sister began to curse the team, telling them to leave. The team did not leave; instead, they asked Mr. and Mrs. B. if they preferred to have a session without taping it, since it was evident that they had changed their minds. Mr. B. answered that he did not mind having the session taped, but his wife had asked him not to allow it, even though she had already agreed to it. When Mrs. B. heard this, she denied her husband's words. During the argument that ensued, it was clear that the issue had also been discussed with the extended family and that Mrs. B. had been told not to agree to it without some concrete reason, not "just because." The team then suggested to the family that they begin the session without taping it, and they asked Mr. and Mrs. B. if it was possible to meet only with the nuclear family, that is, without Mrs. B.'s sister. The B.s, who perceived the flexibility and understanding of the team, accepted their suggestion. The session began with the family therapist sharing her feeling of how the therapeutic process might be frightening for them, since they did not yet know her well enough, though they knew the case manager. In doing so, she allowed the clients to express their fear; she asked the family if any other situations had required them to make decisions in an environment of fear and uncertainty.

* * *

The ability of the team to interpret the situation as an example of the family reality and to relate to the meaning of the offensive behavior, rather than to the behavior itself, helped them to join the family. When the team had to change their plan to videotape the session after they had specially arranged it and brought all the equipment, they experienced a sense of disorganization and lack of stability. Joining allowed the team to reflect on the experience without judging it or without actually agreeing to it, thus leading the family toward a less disorganized situation.

Some therapists explain this kind of family behavior as resistance and fear of change (Schlosberg and Kagan, 1988). However, from a joining perspective, it is possible to perceive such behavior as the way in which the family communicates to the therapist what it means to live in such a disorganized and unstable reality. It is also an opportunity for the therapist to communicate that it is possible to understand this distress without being threatened by it, thereby beginning the process of creating a supportive therapeutic environment in which the family can learn to trust and feel safe.

When working with FED, it is more accurate to define the tool as "joining and rejoining" (Sharlin and Shamai, 1995). Joining is usually done during the first phase of therapy, and as the intervention proceeds, it becomes a natural part of the process. However, when working with FED, the joining that is done initially does not always suffice for the duration of the intervention. These families, who often have histories of disappointment with previous interventions and of abandonment by the helping professions, are suspicious of any, and all, therapists. Such families are constantly testing therapists to find out whether they can be trusted, and the therapeutic team must invest a lot of time and energy throughout the entire process to rejoin with the family.

Case Illustration

When the team arrived at the home of the S. family for their fourth session, they met Mrs. S. at the entrance, who was about to take her daughter to kindergarten. Mrs. S. was still in her nightgown. When she saw the team, she completely ignored them. D., the family therapist, approached Mrs. S. and told her that she understood the family had just woken up and that it would be difficult to begin treatment immediately; she suggested that the team could wait a while, until the family got organized, or could, if necessary, postpone the meeting until the afternoon. Mrs. S.'s eyes lit up, and she asked the team to wait a few minutes until the family could organize itself. During the session, Mrs. S. was much more cooperative than in previous sessions. It seems that the accepting and caring behavior of the team, along with their respectful attitude toward how the family organizes its time, allowed the continuation of the therapeutic process and even had an effect on the attitude of the family during the session.

* * *

With middle-class populations, a framework of time has to be maintained to increase the effectiveness of intervention (Fischer, 1978; Mallucio and Marlow, 1974; Seabury, 1976; Shamai, 1987). By contrast, therapy with FED calls for different approaches to joining and rejoining with families, even if they violate the therapeutic contract and the creation of boundaries and organization. It is important to remember that our first concern is to ensure that the therapeutic process continues, with the changing of specific behaviors being a secondary focus.

Structuring and Creating Boundaries

Boundaries within FED are targeted toward increasing the organization of the family. These boundaries define roles and relationships within the family and between the family and society. The structure of the intervention is the basis for increasing organization. Besides the specific duration of the intervention, as well as the time and the place of the meetings, there is also a clear and discrete role definition for each team member. Since we are suggesting a multilevel intervention that focuses on the behavioral and emotional functioning of the family, as well as on their financial difficulties and their disconnection from social institutions in the community, the discrete roles of the team members are defined according to the different levels of intervention. The family therapist is responsible for carrying out the therapeutic process; the case manager is responsible for making connections with other social institutions.

Case Illustration

During the second meeting with the S. family, Mr. S. was very depressed. He was afraid of being arrested because he had many debts and the creditors were complaining about it to the police. It seemed that neither Mr. S. nor Mrs. S. could concentrate on the issue. Both of them were interested in working on their relationship, especially the decision Mr. S. had made not to sleep with his wife. The family therapist invited the case manager to take fifteen minutes to explore, together with the family, whether something could be done to prevent Mr. S.'s possible arrest. The case manager asked about the extent of their debt, and she found that part of the debt was the result of purchasing basic needs, such as furniture, appliances, and so on, and that part of it was the result of bad financial management. Since the family had already acquired their basic needs, it was clear that the only way to prevent increasing their debt was to reorganize the family budget. Mr. and Mrs. S. were asked whether they were ready to prepare a list of family income and expenditures and to work together with the case manager toward balancing it. Both of them agreed to it, but indicated that they needed a quick solution to the existing debt. They had already tried using the solution of unified debts,* but the amount set by the judge was too high, and they could not continue payments. The case manager suggested another appeal to the court as the only possible solution, offering a letter from the Department of Social Services that would describe the therapeutic procedure that the family was undergoing. Mr. S. wondered whether the judge would allow a second chance for unified debts and, if so, whether he would be able to pay the amount set by the judge. While expressing his doubts, Mr. S. described the complicated procedure involved in applying for unified debts. It was clear that he was very ambivalent about whether to accept the suggestion of the case manager. When the case manager realized this, she reflected her feeling to Mr. S. and challenged him by asking both Mr. and Mrs. S. whether they could think of another way or whether they had accepted the idea of Mr. S.'s possible arrest. They agreed that the only way to solve the

*This is a legal process used by people who are indebted to many creditors and are unable to pay. They can make a court appeal for combining their debts, and if granted, the judge sets a fixed monthly amount to be repaid, while taking into consideration the financial circumstances of the individual. The money being paid each month is then divided among the creditors proportionately, according to the size of the debt owed to each.

problem was by reappealing to the court and thanked the case manager for her efforts to help them, particularly her letter to the judge. Knowing the disorganization of the family, the case manager set up a meeting with Mr. S., asking him to prepare all the material needed for the appeal to the court. She asked him to specify exactly what was needed and what he was going to do to fulfill those needs.

* * *

During the treatment process, a boundary system is created by defining the rules of the meetings, such as when and how one can speak (Sharlin and Shamai, 1995). The therapist must use concrete terms to explain rules and tasks so that each member of the family can clearly define his or her role. In one case, the therapist used two signals resembling a traffic light to overcome the chaotic behavior of the family members. Each member was allowed to talk only on the green signal.

When creating boundaries to redirect the disorganization toward a more defined and organized lifestyle, the role of each family member must be clearly specified. This has to be undertaken by the therapist in several stages: (1) understanding the disorganization and the way in which it affects the behavior and arouses the feelings of family members, (2) joining with the feelings that are aroused by the disorganized situation, and (3) challenging the family members to work toward overcoming the disorganization by defining their roles and accepting their commitment to implement these roles.

Case Illustration

S., the oldest daughter in a single-parent family, was critical of the way her mother educated her younger brothers; consequently, whenever the mother said something to the boys that S. did not accept, she attempted to intervene. This usually resulted in verbal and physical violence between S. and her mother, while the young boys used this fighting to ignore their mother's request. The therapist realized that S. needed to be recognized as the "older daughter"; however, the price she was paying for it was high, as well as damaging to her own developmental process. Therefore, the family therapist suggested a session with S. and her mother, Mrs. C.:

FT: It seems that there are many incidents of physical and verbal violence between both of you. What is going on?

Mrs. C.: Yes, you are right. Since S. decided to leave the boarding school, life at home has become one long fight. She thinks that she has the right to educate the children and to tell me what to do, how to do it, and the worst—to curse me.

S.: Yes, you are a whore, a bitch; you destroy your kids; you are a bitch . . . [Mrs. C. got up, went to S., and both of them began to hit each other. The family therapist intervened between the two by holding the mother and asking the case manager to hold S. Both mother and daughter continued to verbally attack each other.]

FT: Now quiet, I am talking! We are holding both of you because we don't accept violence inside or outside the session. We would like to find ways to change the unbearable situation for both of you, but we will be able to do it only if each one of you can commit yourself to stopping the verbal and physical violence.

Mrs. C.: I must say that I am no longer going to allow her to talk to me like this. She can leave home; no one needs her there. She is terrorizing everyone, including her brothers and sisters.

S.: Shut up, bitch.

FT: Mrs. C., can you do something about this situation?

Mrs. C.: Yes. It can't go on like this. She has to understand that I am the mother at home.

S.: What mother . . .

FT: S., now it's between myself and your mother. [To the case manager] Please, can you hug her and help her to be quiet while I am talking to her mother? [To Mrs. C.] Now, let me understand exactly what is going on at home.

Mrs. C.: Since S. left the boarding school, life at home has become unbearable. She intervenes between me and the boys, and everyone feels terrorized by her. She told me that she left the boarding school so she could take care of and educate her brothers. No one wants her to do it. She is a teenager; she has her school and her friends. I give her pocket money to go out with her friends and to behave like a girl her age. She is not a mother. You know, she looks at TV soap operas and demands another house and new furniture and begins to curse when I tell her that I don't have money for it.

FT: So, there is a fight about the mother's role at home.

Mrs. C.: Yes. She always tries to tell me what to do, and I wish we would have nice relations, like girlfriends, so she could tell me things that relate to her age.

FT: Maybe part of the problem is that you confuse S. when you say you want her as a girlfriend. She is your daughter, and these are completely different roles. I wonder, how can you keep your role as a mother and at the same time be a friend to S.?

Mrs. C.: Maybe friend is not the right word. I would like us to have a close relationship. When I was a teenager, I was always afraid of my parents. I respected them and loved them, but I wanted to be able to share things with them. Now, I wish my daughter could do that with me.

FT: So, you want S. to feel and behave like a girl who is seventeen years old and to be able to share things with you. In my experience, teenagers often like "to teach" their parents what is "good parenting." I wonder how you can allow S. to do that without giving up your role as a mother and the one who is responsible for raising and educating S. and the other children?

Mrs. C.: Well, this is difficult. I don't believe S. will let me do it; she always—

FT: Let's not talk about what S. will let you do and what she won't. Let's talk about your role, your responsibility, your power.

Mrs. C.: I am not sure that I do have any power at home since S. came back.

S.: She always blames me; you don't have power because you do not deserve it—

Mrs. C.: Shut—

FT: No, this kind of discussion between both of you will not have a place here. In fact, you do not need me to talk like this. You are doing it perfectly, but both of you remain hurt and frustrated. So, let's go back to our main issue. Mrs. C., you wonder about your power; you are afraid you do not have enough power to be the mother of S., but if I remember your history, you are a very brave woman. You raised four young children while holding a job in the hospital as a practical nurse; you had to defend yourself and the children against your husband's physical abuse, and you did it. I even wonder if S. did not learn her assertive behavior from you. Had she another significant woman to learn from?

Mrs. C.: [Smiles] Well, I guess there is something in what you just said. I do know that there were things I did that S. did not like, but she still cannot understand everything. I hope that one day, I will be able to explain to her; maybe you would help me. But I do not accept her attitude toward me and her siblings; her behavior cannot continue for even one hour more.

FT: So, what do you want to do about it?

Mrs. C.: I won't let S. talk to me like she used to. When she starts, I will ask her to stop or to leave the house until she calms down. I am ready to listen to her, to explain to her my view of things, but I am not ready to let her hurt me or the children or for her to act like a queen. [Mrs. C. talked in a quiet and assertive voice, and S. began to cry.] [To S.] I love you, and I really respect your motivation in school, your intelligence, but you are only a teenager, you are not yet a mother; enjoy your time, enjoy your friends, and don't try to compete with me; this won't work.

S.: [Crying] You are right, but I really care about my brother and sister and I can't forgive you for working as an escort woman. I wonder whether you can educate us after what you have done.

Mrs. C.: Again, you are trying to educate me. We can talk about my job at the office. I was not an escort woman, but you will have to stop relating to me like shit. I won't let you continue with it. You want to take care of your brother and sister, but, in fact, you are a very bad model for them. This is not the way a child should behave. Would you like your children to relate to you like this?

FT: It seems to me that you really do have power; you were very assertive, you explained yourself very clearly, and it seems to me that you touched S.'s feelings and thoughts. How can you continue with this behavior at home? How can you respect yourself and your daughter so that you can keep this power?

Mrs. C.: This will be difficult; you can encourage me, but you are not living with us.

S.: [Laughs sarcastically] Ask M. [the family therapist] for a picture so you can remember her and what she said.

FT: There is something in what you said. We sometimes use these kinds of "tricks" to help remind people of things. Do you have another idea on how to remind you and your mother about what was done here besides a picture, since I don't have one [with a smile]?

S.: This is funny and ridiculous. She will remember.

FT: I am not so sure that under a stressful situation, you will remember it.

Mrs. C.: Well, S. can remind me.

FT: Oh no, this is your responsibility to maintain your role and status as a mother, and I guess that S., like many other teenagers, expects you to have this role even though she fights and criticizes it.

S.: It is not exactly like that. I think—

FT: S., our issue now is a mother's role, and it is between me and your mother. I really understand your concern about your mother and your efforts to help her when I challenge her, but I'm sure that she can cope with it.

Mrs. C.: Yes, and in fact, I am still thinking about something that can help me remember our discussion today. I guess I learned something today about my relationship with S. . . . Maybe I can write on a piece of paper the sentence "I am the mother here" and put it on the refrigerator.

FT: This is wonderful.

S.: This is silly.

Mrs. C.: No, it is not!

Structuring and creating boundaries are tools that touch the core of the problems of the FED population. Many of the actual problems presented by these families are typical of the nuclear structure of the family and the respective roles of family members. Therefore, when working toward creating boundaries and role definitions, the therapist must consider that beyond the apparent problems, there are painful questions nagging the family members: Who can assume the given role (whatever it may be)? Can I, he, or she, cope with it? What is going to happen if the member who is responsible for it will not accept it?

When working with the FED population, the fundamental requirement of the therapist and/or the team is to take responsibility for the therapeutic context. It is often unrealistic to expect the family to be responsible for the therapeutic context, especially in the first phase of treatment. With our client population, it was the case manager who called families to remind them about meetings or to find out whether they had completed a task that they had been assigned. Although this could be perceived as condescending, and therefore disrespectful of the family, we view it as a demonstration of real concern and understanding of the families' problems and as a means of overcoming many situations that would otherwise end either in termination or avoidance of treatment due to an alleged lack of motivation.

In any case, creating boundaries and structure is better accomplished by the team through the use of tools such as empowerment and suggestive techniques rather than by giving "orders." When trying to achieve a lasting outcome, it is important to help the family grow by developing each member's potential skills to create and change the family's structure and boundaries according to different life phases and unexpected situations. Since this kind of flexibility requires a strong self-image, other goal-oriented techniques employing narrative, empowerment, and communication skills are used. However, goal-oriented techniques can be used effectively only when the therapeutic system is perceived as a secure context for the family, and only after intensive use of the preparatory techniques described in this chapter.

Chapter 6

Expanding the Toolbox: Using Goal-Oriented Techniques

This chapter will focus on describing the goal-oriented techniques aimed at creating a specific change in the family. However, it is important to mention again that it is often impossible to fully distinguish between all other preparatory techniques and goal-oriented ones, and in many cases, they may overlap. For example, creating structure and boundaries might be perceived as a preparatory technique that enables the family to use therapy, as well as a goal-oriented technique directed toward changing the family structure. Usually what is being done in the two cases is quite similar, with the differences being expressed in the defined goal of using the technique. We will describe two main goal-oriented techniques: (1) empowering techniques, which include suggestive techniques, reframing, re-authoring life narratives, and written messages; and (2) enhancing communication skills, which enables direct and clear communication in a respectful way, helping to maintain family boundaries and structure.

EMPOWERING TECHNIQUES

Before describing empowering techniques, it is important to clarify the term. The linguistic definition of the term empowering is to give power or authority. This definition implies the hierarchical relationship between the therapist and the family. It often puts the therapist in a position of "knowing" what is good for the family and how it should function. Looking at the history of interventions with poor and disorganized families, we can find many cases that assume this kind of attitude, beginning with the "friendly visitors" (Bruno, 1948) and continuing in projects that are being implemented even today (Aram).

The attractiveness of this kind of intervention is that one can present a defined goal and technique that are often accepted by societal institutions, such as the welfare, health, and educational systems. However, it leaves the family in a position of powerlessness, as if its members cannot define and make decisions about their own lives. However, the term empowerment can also be used to describe a dialogue between the family and the therapist through which the family is continuously supported in developing as many opportunities as possible that seem appropriate for fulfilling the family's needs. Creating a dialogue means that the therapist accepts the fundamental supposition that if the family has survived up to this point, then some skills must have been acquired and used by family members, even though this is not always obvious to the family. The role of the therapist is, therefore, to include the family in a mutual process in which family skills are discovered and acknowledged, thus reawakening hope and enhancing the ability of the family to overcome the present distress.

There are a variety of means to empower a family in extreme distress, such as focusing on certain family strengths of which the therapist is aware, as in the case of the L. family: "Maybe you do not appreciate it enough, but the fact that you, the parents, could organize this meeting and take responsibility for all your children showing up, illustrates your competence as organizers of the family, the respect you get from your children, who were ready to invest time in a family meeting, and your deep concern about things that are happening in the family." (See Chapter 8 for a more in-depth look at the L. family.) This kind of focusing is often done by the therapist to support and enhance the family's strength. However, it should be emphasized that whenever this tool is used, it must be based on the honest perception of the therapist. "As if" behavior of the therapist, which evolves from knowing that it is helpful to support strength, is often perceived by the family as artificial and can be counterproductive, resulting in lowered self-esteem among family members. In such cases, families feel that they are so weak that the therapist must use any available ploy to show them something positive.

Suggestive Techniques

Suggestive techniques refer to the process of bringing an idea to mind through association with other ideas that are meaningful to the individual and to the family. The use of suggestive techniques has been an integral part of therapeutic interventions, without referring to these techniques directly or explicitly. The influence of suggestion appears in the literature in two main areas: its effect on the results of treatment and its use in therapists' messages to families.

The first area examines the influence of suggestion on the results of treatment, with special attention devoted to studying the placebo effect in different populations. Many studies show that positive change can occur without actually giving treatment, but rather by building a set of expectations that something—not necessarily therapy—will help (Shapiro and Morris, 1978). According to many studies, about 33 percent of the positive results of treatment seem to be related to the placebo effect, which is created by the expectations of the clients (Bergin and Lambert, 1978). If so, then building expectations at the beginning of the intervention should be an integral and important ingredient when clients are being prepared for therapy. When working with families in extreme distress who have had painful experiences with social service departments, mental health services, and educational authorities, building a set of hopeful expectations is extremely important. In the project discussed in this book, the families were told about the project by their social workers, who presented it as a "very special project" run by "very experienced family therapists," with the families having been "chosen" to take part in the project. We believe that each service agency can create some "special attractions" to create hopeful expectations for the family as a basis for trust, such as supervision or consultation by an expert, a special new program, and so forth. It is important, however, that such "attractions" be honored.

The second area of suggestion focuses on messages presented by therapists to the families during treatment. These are usually verbal messages, which are perceived by the clients on a conscious level, known as the "representational system," as well as on an unconscious level, called the "reference system." The integration between the representational system and the reference system affects the "lead system," which is used to decide whether and how to accept conveyed information (Bandler and Grinder, 1979). In analyzing the therapeutic sessions that were conducted in this project, it was obvious that many suggestive messages were being used, either to join the family or to create some changes in family members' attitudes and behaviors.

Case Illustration

In the third meeting with the J. family, Mr. J. told the team that when their neighbors found out about their involvement in a special welfare project, they suggested making a mess in the house to create the impression that they needed additional financial aid. He added that he could not accept his neighbors' advice since a clean and aesthetic home was very important to him. The therapist picked up on this point and used it to reinforce Mr. J.'s sense of pride and self-esteem:

> **FT:** Yes, we can see how much you invest in your home and how you decorate it with your artistic handicrafts.
>
> **Mr. J.:** Yes, I love my home, and I love to take care of it. I also like to make artistic handicrafts to decorate the house.
>
> **FT:** This is wonderful. You are a very unique person. Not many husbands are willing to invest as much in their homes, and sometimes, even if they do so, they would not admit it, since they do not consider this masculine behavior. You are quite special, creative, caring, and brave.

The next meeting took place about one month later. When the team arrived, the J. family reported that meaningful changes had occurred during the past month. Mr. and Mrs. J. decided that they needed to improve their financial situation. Since Mrs. J. was getting better with people and with taking "orders" from "managers," she would be the one to go out to work, while Mr. J. would take on the household responsibilities and the children's education:

FT: This is wonderful—

Mrs. J.: [Entered in the middle, telling about her success at work]

FT and Team: [Encouraged and supported her]

Mr. J.: I think that I deserve some support and encouragement also. She can go to work and enjoy it because she knows that I can be trusted and that everything at home will be perfect. I don't think many men would do such a thing.

Mrs. J.: Yes! You are right, you really help, and I can really trust you.

It seems that the message transmitted in the previous meeting affected the family's "lead system" and helped family members to be proud of their uniqueness and to perceive this as a power that could be used to open new alternatives for coping with a bad financial situation. Here we would like to emphasize the underlying danger of suggestive techniques. The temptation to use suggestive messages with FED is very high. In their disorganized way of life, such messages can generate a degree of certainty about the effectiveness of treatment and can give the therapist a sense of control in situations that would resemble anarchy to someone outside the family system (Amundson, Stewart, and Valentine, 1993; Atkinson, 1993). Many interventions with FED are also done under court order (i.e., as an outcome of violence, child abuse, or as a condition to removing the child from the home). In such situations, the therapist has to be even more sensitive to the power exercised over the family. Therefore, suggestive messages should be used in a form that will lead to a dialogue in which the family has an option to either reject the message, ignore it, reframe it, or accept only part of it.

Reframing

Minuchin and Fishman (1981) define reframing as a clash between the way in which the family perceives and frames reality and the way in which the therapist perceives reality. Presenting the therapist's reality to the family introduces other alternatives for new modes of thinking and behaving.

Case Illustration

The L. family had eleven children. The oldest one died at the age of seven, after a severe illness, and four of the other ten children were either in foster homes or in boarding schools. The parents had a strong feeling of failure in relation to rearing and educating their children. They were, therefore, very anxious and resentful when their teenage daughter, G., wanted to leave home and go to a boarding school. She was supported by her teachers, which increased the parents' anxiety and aggressive attitude toward all social institutions. When they met with the therapeutic team and expressed their anger about the situation, the family therapist responded by reframing their definition of "good parents" and "bad parents":

> As I hear your pain and anger, I wonder what exactly causes this pain. I think it has to do with the fact that one of your children is staying with a foster family and another three are at boarding school. In fact, I think that you are good parents. You are the kind of parents who see what is good for your children. You will do what's good for your children even if it is very difficult for you, and that means that you are good parents. It was difficult for you to send your daughter to live with a foster family, but it happened because you, Mrs. L., were sick when your daughter was very young and neither you nor Mr. L., who was taking care of you and the other children, could look after her. Your daughter adjusted very well to the foster family and remained there while maintaining close contact with you. It required a strong and caring attitude to give up your natural desire for the benefit of your daughter. The same was true with the other three children. Sending them to a boarding school means understanding that these schools can give them the best conditions for using and enhancing their abilities. Again, you put your own needs behind those of your children. I think this makes you very good parents.

This message was accepted by the parents because it related to the family's perception of "good" and "bad," but reframed its definition, reducing the parents' anxiety and anger and making them calmer in their relationship with their teenage daughter. After hearing the reframing, G., herself, began to perceive her parents as caring and, by the end of the treatment, was no longer asking to leave home. She described changes at home, especially in the way that her parents functioned. This helped her to enhance her communication with both parents, especially with her mother, which was important for her when discussing gender-related issues. (The full therapeutic process with the L. family is described in Chapter 8.)

* * *

When working with families in extreme distress, reframing should be strongly based on the subjective reality of the family. Through reframing, the therapist suggests another subjective reality, without ignoring the family's perception of its reality, and thereby provides the family with another option.

Reauthoring Life Narratives

Life narratives have been used in family therapy from a variety of theoretical perspectives. One of these focuses on the meaning of the story while trying to challenge this meaning through cognitive or behavioral approaches. This way of using life narratives is often employed by structural therapists (Minuchin and Fishman, 1981), strategic therapists (Haley, 1976; Madanes, 1981), and systemic therapists, especially the Milan group. During the last decade, the use of narratives in family therapy has been strongly connected with the postmodern perspective (Parry and Doan, 1994; White 1990; White and Epston, 1989; White, 1995). It follows on the understanding that since there is no single universal truth, any one way in which people interpret their lives is valid and has special meaning for the interpreter. In working with FED, this perspective has particular relevance, since most of the families have a long history with social agents from different institutions who have tried to judge and invalidate their interpretations, trying "to educate" them with the "right meanings."

When using narratives with a family in extreme distress, it is important to first give the family the opportunity to tell its story and just to listen and to explore that story's meaning. Telling the family's story in front of an audience, that is, to the therapeutic team and other family members, serves to validate the story. The interest and understanding expressed by the therapeutic team often enhances the self-esteem of the family, as indicated by Mr. C.: "to talk with you [referring to the therapeutic team] was different; it was not like with friends in the neighborhood. . . ." When this atmosphere of trust is created, the therapist can further explore by asking questions that reveal additional information, thereby widening the meaning of the story and, in effect, reauthoring the story in such a way that it opens alternatives for the family.

Case Illustration

N. was the oldest teenage daughter in her family; she had three younger sisters and a brother. Their mother, who had divorced her husband about four years before applying for therapy, was raising the children. The reason for the divorce was the husband's violent behavior toward his wife and children, as well as his drinking problem. N.'s mother, who was known at the Department of Social Services, asked for help with N., with whom she had had many conflicts, as N. had tried to assume her missing father's role and "to educate the entire family."

In meetings with the family, N. expressed anger toward her parents, especially her father. At one meeting, when she talked about school, she mentioned her keen interest in Bible studies, which are an integral part of the educational program in Israel:

> **FT:** How do you explain this interest you have in the Bible?
>
> **N.:** This is because of my dad. When I was little, he used to sit with me and tell me stories from the Bible, and I liked them very much.
>
> **FT:** Well, this is very interesting. It's the first time you are introducing me to this side of your dad.
>
> **N.:** Yes. I always talk about his faults, but this is not the entire story. I think he also cared about us. He bought our apartment; he read to me when I was a child, and I think that I like to study because of him. It is very sad to see how he became a heavy drinker. I feel very sorry for him, though I cannot help him.

During that week, N. visited her father. A week later she invited her brother and sisters to accompany her and asked her mother whether she would agree to bake a cake or cookies for their father. This became a regular weekly visit by the children, and the mother even cooperated by sending something she had cooked for their father. On one occasion, when they found the father drunk, N. was very angry and disappointed and took her siblings back home. It was the mother who reminded her "that there are different sides to her father, as she had expressed in therapy, and that the next visit could be more successful." N. smiled and continued the contact between herself, her siblings, and their father. Accepting the father as not "totally bad" diminished her need to replace his role in the family, thus reducing conflicts between her and her mother. This also affected the mother's life story, and her cooperation with the children's desire to meet with their father helped to reduce tensions at home. The young brother even expressed pride in "having a father who knows how to tell stories." It seems that the family members enriched their meaning of "good" and "bad" when relating to the father.

Written Messages

Written messages were originally used by the Milan team at the end of each meeting (Tomm, 1984). In our project, a written message was given to the family only at the last meeting, along with a painting illustrating the written message. The written message is something concrete—a letter that can be read and reread—and a painting can be hung on the wall as a constant reminder. Most of the families were excited to receive the message; some said they would put it in their bedrooms so they would see it every day. It seems that combining the concrete level with the cognitive level was useful to FED, who often tend to relate to complicated events on a very concrete level. The written messages summarize the narrative of the family story, as told by the family, including metaphors that either were used by the family during the sessions or were offered by the therapeutic team and accepted by the family. Particular emphasis is placed on the words and descriptions that open new alternatives for the family in terms of coping strategies and behaviors. The message is first read by the team and then presented to the family.

Case Illustration

The following written message was given to the S. family by the team at their last meeting:

Dear S. (Mrs. S.) and C. (Mr. S.),

It seems to us that after ten meetings, we can summarize and evaluate part of the treatment and find out what was learned during the process that can be available and useful to you in your everyday life. In our meetings, we focused on your family and your relationship. We realized very readily that the main theme in your relationship is love. Each of you has strong feelings toward the other, and both of you trust each other. The love and the trust have been built through the years of being together. C., your love for S. is expressed by your appreciation of her and recognition of her honesty, her dedication, and her tendency to have a pessimistic view of life. S., your love for C. is expressed by your appreciation of his honesty, loyalty, sense of humor, and optimistic ideas. Your love is your strength. You are very strong. You have the strength to build together, and you have the strength to destroy together [repeating the word strength many times is a suggestive technique].

Through your love, you have built many things in your relationship: you overcame the difficulties in getting pregnant; you overcame the difficulties during pregnancy; you are trying to cope with three babies and financial difficulties, and supporting each other during the time C. has been trying to stop drinking. Both of you admit that you would be able to cope with all the difficulties through mutual support. But with your strength, you also have the ability to destroy. When your relationship begins to deteriorate, you are like a driver who loses the brakes of his car in the middle of a mountain slope. [Since Mr. S. is the driver, this metaphor is used for a suggestive goal.] Then you are crossing the red line by blaming and humiliating each other, and even by using physical violence. Sometimes it seems that you have not yet found the way to feel your love during the routine of everyday life. You need the excitement, the high volume, and then you either love or hate each other.

What worries us is that in this situation, you lose the loyalty to each other and become loyal to the "institution of marriage." Loyalty to the institution of marriage weakens your relationship. When both of you choose to become loyal to the institution of marriage, then C. is loyal to his family of origin and S. is loyal to her family of origin. The values of your family, C., require the wife to act according to her husband's demands. The wife must always be loyal and respectful to her husband, without raising doubts or questions. In your family, S., you have learned that the woman is always a victim of her husband and that the man is the one to blame for it. In your family, intimacy did not exist and secrets were told without regard for boundaries. Keeping these values of the families of origin prevents you from building your family as a "common business." Only when you decide to choose, either in building or in destroying, will you be able to commit yourself to the choice. You have developed a special skill to hurt each other, and in so doing, you also hurt yourselves. When C. is hurt, he usually turns to the bottle and drinking. He then becomes soft, without boundaries and without "brakes" when driving [here again relating to C.'s world]. When S. is hurt, she usually experiences an asthma attack, she does not have enough air, her body becomes tense and rigid, and she becomes the "brakes."

But, each one of you also has special skills in being dedicated and committed. S. is committed to the housework and to educating and caring for the children. C. is dedicated to his job. We think that it is the right time for each of you to invest in your growth. If you do it, then you, C., would be able to learn from S. about how to be sometimes tough like "fimo" [a hard plastic that was used as a metaphor], and S. would have the chance to learn from C. about how to be sometimes soft like Play-Doh. In both of you, we can find the toughness and the softness. We, the team, must trust your experience in being committed to each other. If you choose to use this commitment, then you will have many chances to complement each other and to use the phrase you often used during treatment: "You were great."

In a follow-up that was done a few years after the therapy ended, we found that the messages and the painting illustrating the messages had been kept and were used by the family (see Chapter 12).

ENHANCING COMMUNICATION SKILLS

During the 1960s and 1970s, studies indicated that low verbal communication is often characteristic of multiproblem FED (Polansky et al., 1970; Polansky, 1971; Polansky, Borgman, and DeSaix, 1972; Polansky, DeSaix, and Sharlin, 1972). It is important to indicate that in the 1990s, we might find richer verbal communication within FED, mostly due to heavy exposure to television. However, this communication is usually nondirect, consisting of conflicting messages often expressed in violent terms. The lack of adequate communication skills, such as listening and being congruent or consistent, prevents direct and clear communication among family members. In working on issues of communication during the therapeutic session, the family is able to experience some benefit from listening and being listened to and can thus realize the importance of direct and clear communication in daily family functioning. By focusing on communication skills, the therapist is able to reinforce verbal, direct, and clear messages, while limiting the type of communication that amplifies violence and alienation through expressions of fear, anxiety, pain, and anger. Techniques such as modeling and role-playing are used in building communication skills, followed by intensive support from the therapist.

Case Illustration

The Z. family was looking for a way to convince their son, L., to go back to school. L. had been absent from school for almost three months:

> **FT:** As you decided in our last meeting, we should try today to help L. return to school. Since all the family members know what school is, and some of the members have also experienced situations of missing school, it is important that all of

you are here. [To the father] I think that you, as the father of the family, should open the discussion. I would like you to turn to L. and ask him about his difficulties in going back to school.

Father: [To the therapist] The problem is that L. is very young and not a smart boy. He tries to imitate his brother A. [who dropped out of school]. I tried to explain to him in a nice way, I beat him, and nothing helped.

FT: [To the father] School is sometimes a very frightening place for young children. [To the other children in the family] What do you think, is it difficult in school?

The other children in the family joined the family therapist and said that it was very difficult in school with their studies, teachers, and friends:

L.: Once I even cried in school because I did not have a friend.

FT: [Returning to the father] Please talk with him. Please try, if only for our discussion. You can ask, "L., what is difficult for you in school?" [Here, the therapist acted as a model.]

Father: [To the therapist] Please leave it. I have already talked with him. There is nothing more to do.

FT: I know that it is very difficult to speak with a young child. But I am sure that even young children have an opinion. Would you like to try to find out whether your child has an opinion? [Here the therapist tried to challenge the father to talk directly with his son.]

Father: L., what's so hard for you in school?

L.: I am embarrassed to go to the new school.

Father: Would you rather go to your old school?

This was the basis for opening a direct discussion between the father and his son. The therapist gave an enormous amount of support and verbal reinforcement to the father for his goodwill in trying to understand L. As the session continued, the father tried to explain the reasons for L.'s embarrassment:

FT: So, L. is embarrassed. [To L.] Who in your family is a specialist in embarrassment?

L.: G. [His brother, sixteen years old and a very quiet boy]

G.: [Smiles]

FT: [To L.] If G. is the specialist in being embarrassed, please consult with him on how to get along in the new school. You are right about being embarrassed in a new place, and it is very important to know how to get along with a feeling of embarrassment. Since G. is a specialist in embarrassment, he is the one to consult.

L.: [Quiet, does not answer]

Father: Answer her already [rushing him].

FT: [To the father] Please, don't rush him. It is very difficult to know how to ask directly. [The therapist identified with the father's difficulty, while at the same time she gave a clear boundary to the father as well as a model for how the father could understand his children and respect them.] [To L.] G. is the one who knows best in your family how to be embarrassed, and he is the one to talk with about embarrassment. You can't consult with someone who doesn't know how to be embarrassed and how to live with it.

L.: [To G.] How can I live with it?

G.: [Quiet, does not answer]

Father: Answer him . . .

G.: [To the therapist] He doesn't have to be embarrassed. All his friends are in school.

FT: [To G.] Please, don't talk to me; talk directly to L., one man to another. Tell him: Don't be embarrassed. You have friends there . . .

G.: [To L.] Don't be embarrassed in school. All your friends are there.

L.: But I am embarrassed.

G.: By whom?

L.: By the new teacher.

G.: But there are many friends from the neighborhood and from the club in school.

L.: It's the new teacher and the new friends, and lots of friends I used to meet at the club aren't coming to the club anymore.

G.: Well, it will take time, but you will get used to the teacher and to the friends. First of all, try to get along with those whom you already know and only later with new friends.

Since the family therapist persisted and would not give up during this session, the family members finally succeeded in communicating directly. It is important to indicate that our intention is not to teach the family communication skills, as suggested in behavioristic approaches to family therapy (Stuart, 1980). Basing our philosophy on the fact that FED already have some communication skills, our goal is to help the family create a context within which these skills can be expressed. As illustrated in the previous case, it is the dialogue with the family that creates the space for its members to listen and express ideas and feelings, as well as to discuss and solve problems. Therefore, we see communication not as an end in itself but rather as a means for decision making and problem solving, which constitute the core of family functioning.

Focusing on communication skills requires sensitivity on the part of the therapist for the way the family uses language. On the one hand, the family's way of communicating is due to its cultural and ethnic background, while on the other, it is part of the specific culture created within the family in its everyday relations. When referring to the cultural and ethnic aspects of the language used by the family, it is useful to listen to the way in which language is being used. Some ethnic groups, such as the Ethiopians, use metaphors and stories, whereas Westerners are more down-to-earth. Conversations with the former are usually longer, with numerous idioms, metaphors, and stories through which the subject is understood and discussed. It is therefore imperative that the therapist listens carefully to the stories or metaphors, and when challenging the family's communications skills, its language should be taken into consideration. A very good example is the Ethiopian families' "coffee ritual." One of the rules among the immigrant Ethiopian community in Israel is that every morning the wife prepares coffee for her husband, as a symbol of her obedience. Most Ethiopian women, as immigrants, adjusted much faster than their husbands to the Israeli culture. They learned the Hebrew language better than the men, found jobs, and became financially supportive, while at the same time enjoying the freedoms that women have in Western societies. This development was very threatening to many of the husbands and caused conflicts between spouses. Ki-Tov and Ben David (1993) described an intervention with an Ethiopian couple who shared their marital conflict problems with the social worker. One reason for the conflict was the wife's resistance to offering the morning coffee to her husband. The social worker asked the couple whether preparing coffee has special meaning for the family and was told about the Ethiopian custom. The worker suggested to the family that they continue the ritual, but with some changes. She suggested that the wife prepare coffee for her husband and for herself and that they sit down and drink the coffee together and discuss their experiences from the previous day, for about fifteen minutes, sharing their frustrations, anger, pain, and surprises, as well as their moments of happiness. This was accepted by both spouses, in part because of the social worker's demonstrated sensitivity toward their culture, their interpretations, and their personal pain.

As previously mentioned, the family's language is also influenced by the specific culture that has developed within the family. Being aware of this specific culture is a way of joining with the family, as well as providing a means for creating change. Some families use many aggressive expressions, metaphors, and idioms, whereas other families use vague language to express their fears, uncertainty, and difficulty in making commitments, and still others may use language that focuses on sadness. Since language is often connected to life meanings and ways of thinking, it provides a means of becoming closer to the families through trying to understand what has created their specific use of language. In some cases, for which the use of this type of language limits communication alternatives, it is useful to enrich families' vocabularies with words and metaphors that will provide new alternatives. This can be achieved by direct communication with families, as well as through modeling, interpreting, and reframing. It is through language that therapists can express sensitivity for their clients' cultural and personal needs, show their respect, and achieve greater closeness with their clients by sharing their pain.

USING THE THERAPEUTIC TEAM

The way in which family therapists use the team approach can also be considered an important "tool" or technique that enriches and contributes to the therapeutic process. As described in previous chapters, the main goals of the therapeutic team are (1) to avoid entering into a coalition of despair with FED, thereby enhancing the potential for continuing the therapeutic process, and (2) to create clear-cut roles and a defined structure for team members, thereby preventing possible disorganization among team members as they attend to the various tasks in the process of intervention with FED.

It is noteworthy that the different roles of the team members do not prevent them from acting as cotherapists whenever necessary. As cotherapists, the team members discuss and negotiate among themselves in front of the family. This negotiation not only exposes the family to different ways of thinking and problem solving; sometimes, the opposing assessments of the team put the family members in a paradoxical situation that challenges them to generate their own solution. It is also possible that by joining with at least one of the ideas expressed by the team, the resistance of family members is lowered (Boscolo et al., 1987; Tomm, 1984). This enables negotiating and problem solving that involves each family member listening to the ideas of the others and responding in a respectful way, without resorting to physical violence or psychological abuse.

Case Illustration

During therapy meetings, Mr. L. expressed his anger toward his teenage daughter because she shaved her legs. When Mr. L. was asked how he knew this, he said that his daughter had told his wife, and she had let him know about it. The therapist, who was a mother of two teenage girls herself, turned to another member in the team, who was a father of two teenage girls, and asked whether he, as a father, was used to interfering in feminine matters in his family. The therapist added that in her family, feminine issues were her responsibility. The male therapist concurred that in his family, the teenage girls usually turned to his wife with feminine concerns. If his wife chose to share some of the issues with him, he listened and expressed his point of view. However, it was clear that his responsibility was to reinforce the trust that the girls had in their mother and to let his wife handle it. The female therapist challenged Mr. L. to control himself in the future if his wife were to tell him something about their teenage daughter.

* * *

It was concluded, after analyzing the process, that the different types of communication among team members were very effective in containing the family and in bringing about desired changes. We therefore highly recommend teamwork, in spite of the additional cost. It seems to us that an effective process of intervention, even though more expensive, will be less costly in the end than the endless process of repeated interventions that traditionally have been used with FED.

SUMMARY

The toolbox consists of many techniques. The more varied they are, the more families can benefit from them. It should be remembered that when using these techniques, the therapist has to take into account elements such as gender, race, and ethnic diversity. The therapist has to listen to the special and unique voice of each family as the best guide for choosing the appropriate technique. We would like to suggest a postmodern approach when referring to techniques, namely, that there are no right or wrong techniques, that there is not one uniform goal or only one true means of achieving it. Rather, it is a joint effort in which the therapeutic team and the family try to elaborate and make room for different perceptions, situations, and experiences. Within the framework of the family, as in an orchestra, the dialogue between the musicians and the conductor, as well as the sensitivity of the conductor to the individual instruments, is crucial to creating the unique gestalt of the music.

Chapter 7

Beyond the Therapy Room

No man is an island, entire of itself; every man is a piece of the continent. . . .

John Donne

This quotation may serve as a motto for this chapter to best express the importance of networking. Our biggest enemy is loneliness (Polansky et al., 1981). This is especially true for FED, as they tend to isolate themselves from their environment and specifically avoid ongoing contacts with agencies and formal organizations in their communities. It is our intention to describe here the kind of network that has been an integral part of every intervention with FED, as we have found this to be a necessary factor in working with these families.

In discussing what is a functioning or a nonfunctioning family, Satir (1972) prefers to distinguish between "nourished" and "non-nourished" families. She suggests four major areas that are most essential to describing families. Each of these areas is on a bipolar continuum. The first one is self-worth, which can be either high, consistent with feelings of integrity, honesty, responsibility, compassion, and love, or low, indicative of feeling defeated, desperate, and so forth. The second is communication, which may be either direct or indirect. The third area consists of the rules which exist in every family and which can be either rigid or flexible and changeable. The last area relates to the idea that every family is part of a community that provides institutions and organizations to help individuals and families to function. Only through direct and open relationships within the family, as well as between the family and its environment, can families remain nourished and healthy. By avoiding contact and harboring feelings of fear and hostility, the family disassociates itself from the environment, gradually depriving itself of important resources and becoming "nonnourished."

In following the systemic approach, family therapists adopt the belief that symptoms carried by the individual result from, or are maintained by, systemic interfamilial relationships that are affected by interaction and communication among family members. Hence, to help the individual family member, representing the symptom carrier (or the IP [identified patient]), we need to enlist the cooperation of the entire family. This systemic perspective goes a step further. When a family needs to be helped, we sometimes have to involve the larger system to which the family belongs, which may include members of the extended family, employers, and representatives from all organizations and services in the community where the family resides.

A distinctive feature in working with FED is that therapy involves multiple agencies and services because of the many problems that these families face, requiring the use of multiprofessional teamwork as well. Since in many cases the relationships between the families and these agencies are either impaired, nonexistent, or lacking in ongoing communication, the families may not be fully aware of their rights and therefore do not make effective use of the services available to them. Moreover, they may not even realize that they are eligible to receive such services. The result is that they usually "fall between the cracks." We believe that it is the responsibility of social services departments to take the initiative and show leadership in assisting these families to obtain and take full advantage of the services to which they are entitled. It is here that the case manager can step in and establish multiprofessional teamwork. In cases in which families begin the therapeutic process in institutions, such as health agencies, mental health agencies, or probation services, it is useful at that point for the therapist to initiate a relationship between the family and the social services department. This should help make available as many alternatives as possible for the types of help needed. In most cases, it is suggested that the case manager be the person developing the multiprofessional team; this person should also lead and take responsibility for its operation. Let us begin our discussion with some basic knowledge and skills needed for using a multiprofessional team for interventions with FED.

MULTIPROFESSIONAL TEAMWORK

Ducanis and Golin (1979, p. 3) define multiprofessional teamwork as "a functioning unit, composed of individuals with varied and specialized training, who coordinate their activities to provide services to a client or group of clients."

Multiprofessional teamwork has been referred to differently by a variety of writers. Some prefer to call it simply "teamwork" (Brill, 1976), others refer to it as forming an "interdisciplinary team" (Ducanis and Golin, 1979), and still others refer to it as "collaboration." A voluminous literature has been written on multiprofessional teamwork in the last two decades. Today, it is generally known as a "method of intervention" and is widely used in various fields, though not extensively with FED. Multiprofessional teams (MPTs) have been developed within the medical field and are a major tool for case management in many medical centers. In recent years, technology and special fields of expertise in medicine have been developed to the degree that it is simply impossible for one person to comprehend and control all of the required knowledge as it relates to medicine, education, law, community organizations, and family therapy. Hence, a team of different experts is needed. Such is also the case when working with FED.

There are reasons for and against the use of a multiprofessional team, both for the client and the professional system. The rationale for using a multiprofessional team for the client's benefit may be, first of all, to provide a coordinated service, which will avoid duplication. Many of the problems are interdependent and can therefore be treated more effectively in coordination with one another. A systematic approach to problem solving enables us to find better solutions for complicated problems, achieve better insight, and thus find additional opportunities for further problem solving. By having all involved professionals work together, the onus to coordinate among different agencies is shifted from the family to the team, thus improving the chances to implement preventive measures. Communication among the professions can be enhanced, promoting sharing, learning, and, ultimately, more effective practice (Marshall, Person-Shoot, and Winnicott, 1979; McDaniel and Campbell, 1986).

A few points can be made against the use of a multiprofessional team. Sometimes, members of the team may have a destructive influence on others, or they may be too rigid or narrow in their perspective. This attitude can influence all multiprofessional team members and may hinder the client from obtaining better service. In some cases, it can even damage the aspects of service that are effective. In a given multiprofessional team, the higher status of some professionals may overshadow the lower status of other professionals or paraprofessionals, to the extent that lower-status workers may be unable to contribute effectively. Multiprofessional team members may become specialized to the extent that they develop their own language, approach things in a distinct manner, and become preoccupied with themselves. Another point is that responsibility may be too diffused among the various professionals in the multiprofessional team. It may even take a long time to coordinate a meeting to have an in-depth discussion—just for one family. This situation often exists within social services departments, where social workers are overwhelmed by the enormous amount and complexity of cases that need immediate attention.

Ducanis and Golin (1979) present four premises in their definition of the multiprofessional team. The first is that teamwork is an evolutionary process and must therefore have identifiable developmental stages. The second premise is that teamwork can be effective only when it is supported and sanctioned by the environment in which it exists. The third premise maintains that teamwork, as a concept, must be studied, understood, and practiced to realize its potential. The fourth is that teamwork has been practiced since the early 1920s (Ackerly, 1947) and has been successful.

According to these assumptions, a multiprofessional team must be composed of individuals who represent several professions and share a common goal that binds and directs them toward their common aims and tasks. Multiprofessional team members must have strong professional identities, which includes knowledge, values, skills, and defined aims and goals of each member's specialty, thereby promoting mutual respect, flexibility, and the ability to exchange ideas, even when there is disagreement. Such professionals will neither lose their specific aims nor cling rigidly to their professional goals without understanding the complexity of their client system. Each professional in the team should be able to ask herself or himself, "Am I here for a common purpose? What is that purpose?" Each one must have a clear understanding of his or her function in the team, while appreciating and understanding the contribution of the other team members. It is important that professionals be clear about the roles they can perform and whether they are appropriate for the task set up by the team. It is useful that team members ask themselves questions such as the following:

- Am I clear about my own role in the team?
- Am I clear about the roles of others in the MPT?
- Are these roles in conflict, and if so, where?

The multiprofessional team operates best as a close-knit unit with mutual skills, knowledge, and resources and with joint responsibility for the outcome, being highly committed to an objective held in common by each team member. To adjust to a collective process, without ignoring individual professional responsibility, the following questions should be asked:

- Do I agree to the tasks we set for ourselves?
- Have we defined them adequately?

The team must continually evaluate itself by answering additional questions:

- How effective is a multiprofessional team in its ability to operate and manage itself as a team of independent persons?
- Are we able to fulfill our roles?
- Can we measure the outcome of tasks to ascertain that they have been completed?

Finally, it is important to note that members recruited for the team must be allowed to make decisions on behalf of the organizations they represent and, as experts, should not fear possible litigation. It can be concluded that for the multiprofessional team to operate effectively, three conditions must be met: (1) team members must have a cooperative balance, (2) they should represent their professions to the best of their ability, and (3) the multiprofessional team leader should be trained and skilled in democratic management of the group. Therefore, knowledge of group dynamics, leadership, communication and decision-making skills, conflict theory, and conflict resolution are essentials in effective multiprofessional team therapy.*

STAGES IN MULTIPROFESSIONAL TEAM DEVELOPMENT

The evolutionary process of the multiprofessional team includes the following six stages: (1) becoming acquainted, (2) trial and error, (3) collective indecision, (4) crisis, (5) resolution, and (6) team maintenance (Ducanis and Golin, 1979; Lowe and Herranen, 1981). These stages resemble group evolutionary processes. Just as in group evolution, it is often difficult to clearly differentiate between stages, which may sometimes overlap. The duration of each of the stages depends on the personality of the members, the size of the team, and whether the team is composed of members from the same organization or from different fields, who would not have previous experience in working together. In the following material, we shall briefly summarize each stage.

Becoming Acquainted

This is the initial stage in which the individuals enter the team, usually according to the nature of the problem. Each professional representative must be prepared beforehand for two things: first, for the goals, purpose, and process of multiprofessional teamwork and, second, for the relevant material regarding the family. At the first meeting, the case is presented in order to focus on the problem and reach consensus among team members regarding aims and goals. The professionals invited to participate in the multiprofessional

*For further information about the multiprofessional team and its implications in training and education, please see Ryan, 1996, and Waskell, 1996.

team represent a wide range of the professional hierarchy. However, the leader of the team could be anyone from among the team members, provided that he or she was trained for this task. We note that in this "becoming acquainted" phase, individual productivity is high, while team productivity is low.

Trial and Error

This stage may take place during the second or third meeting while there is early awareness of the need to work together. The process of this stage is characterized by testing the boundaries that might cause a role conflict, as expressed by feelings of suspicion, envy, and territoriality. The most common pattern of interaction emerging at this point is pairing off. This is a natural process whereby individuals seek an ally, usually someone who resembles them and who has a compatible personality. Therefore, decisions at this stage may be made either by the multiprofessional team leader or by the members, in pairs or as a group. Low group productivity can still be seen while individual members strive to reach their stated goals.

Collective Indecision

This is usually the result of the team's attempts at avoiding direct conflict to achieve a degree of equilibrium. Boundaries of the group as a team begin to take shape, but decisions are made by default, giving the appearance of shared responsibility. At this stage, there are no group norms; however, there is the beginning of group conformity. Although there is an attraction to being part of the team, this is still accompanied by ambivalence. Productivity at both the individual and group levels remains low. This is a very fragile state and must be discussed with the group.

Crisis

Members recognize this stage to be the last chance for continuation of the group, while taking into account the opportunities and risks presented. The role of leader must be assumed by one of the team members in cases of undefined leadership. In other instances, the group is preoccupied with itself rather than caring for the client or being "client oriented." The group treats negative emotions that surface as priorities, and personality differences take precedence over professional input centered on the client. Individual productivity varies among team members, while group productivity remains low.

Resolution

At this stage, the group attempts to pull together and function as a team. Teamwork characteristics can be noted, such as open communication, shared leadership, and the ability to make decisions and to undertake responsibility. Satisfaction is the predominant emotion, which results from high individual and group productivity. In many cases, this may not only be the peak of achievement but also a stage for departure. At this point, the client system has been helped and there is no further need for the team. Although certain problems can be resolved with short-term teams, more complex problems call for longer-term multiprofessional teams. This is where the sixth and final stage comes in.

Team Maintenance

Each member of the team is now well adjusted to his or her role in accomplishing the planned tasks and fulfilling client needs. Commitment is strong, and teamwork is further progressing. To maintain the team, the leader and team members must understand the group's dynamics.

It is important to point out that the duration of the multiprofessional team may vary. It can be a longitudinal process or a short and focused process, which may last for only one or two meetings. The duration of the process depends upon the client system. In some cases, one or two meetings are sufficient to help the family, whereas other cases may require a longer process. Maintenance may mean meeting in crisis situations only or more regularly. The latter depends on the perception and policy of the organization.

MULTIPROFESSIONAL TEAMWORK INTERVENTION IN THE CASE OF FED

When using a multiprofessional team for intervention with FED, we integrate the different fields of expertise that are required for the intervention, while also opening new alternative means of contact between the family in distress and the professionals and agencies in the community. In observing multiprofessional teamwork interventions, we can see that teamwork operates according to a problem-solving approach, based on assigned tasks. This approach follows a logical flow: from problem to goals, tasks, roles, and interventions, ending with evaluation, follow-up, or replanning. The following is an example of working with an FED case, as illustrated by the R. family.

Case Illustration

The R. family is composed of Mr. R. (age forty-five), Mrs. R. (age forty-two), and their six children (Mrs. R. was pregnant with their seventh child at the time): A., the oldest son, age twenty-two; B., a fifteen-year-old girl; C., a ten-year-old boy; D., an eight-year-old boy; E., a five-year-old girl; and F., a two-year-old boy. The family is a second-generation Department of Social Services client and is known to all department workers, who have been trying to help this family for years with no success.

Mr. R. completed barely six years of schooling before dropping out, and he now has no permanent occupation. He was drafted into the army at age eighteen and was discharged after six months for misconduct, repeated jail terms, and desertion. He worked periodically in the local market, first selling vegetables and then as a porter. He is known as a heavy drinker and smoker, always getting into fights and becoming very violent. For most of his life, he has worked intermittently, and whatever money he earns is spent on drinking and card playing.

Mr. R.'s father was also a client of the Department of Social Services ever since he immigrated to Israel from Morocco. Although devoutly religious, he was generally known as a bully, beating his wife and forcing his son out of the house. Mr. R. felt as if he had been thrown out of his home and was therefore unable to live a decent life, as he said, "I was always in and out of trouble." He was twenty-three years old when he married the girl he had gotten pregnant, who was twenty at the time. It was later that he learned she had mental problems, but he never bothered to find out exactly what she suffered from and why she was always on medication.

Mrs. R. grew up in a home as one of nine children. Her parents neglected her all of her life. She dropped out of school in sixth grade and has never received any kind of training; she is currently a housewife. She was known as a girl in distress, somewhat retarded, and was treated as "mentally ill" but never hospitalized. She was constantly running away from home and being beaten upon returning.

The couple's oldest son, A., spent several short periods in jail for using drugs. He basically raised himself because his mother had four or five miscarriages in between the births of her first three children and so never had time to look after him. Their fifteen-year-old daughter, B., was known as a girl in distress. She attempted suicide several times because her father would not let her out of the house while wearing the short dresses that she liked. He used to call her a whore, and she would run away from home, which would be followed by his finding her, beating her, and bringing her back home. C. and D. were in fourth and second grades in school, respectively, had learning difficulties, and were known for their truancy. E., the five-year-old daughter, was diagnosed as retarded. She and her two-year-old sister clung to their mother at home and in the streets.

A brief look at the family revealed a very gloomy and hopeless one. Their caseworker described them as "hard to reach, without any motivation to change, in fact, nothing can be done with them." This family was selected as FED according to the research criteria. No one really knew the whole story of the family, but it was obvious that such a family could not be treated and helped unless therapy went "beyond the therapy room." A multiprofessional team seemed to us a necessity from the very first contact.

Mr. R. told the family therapist that he could take care of his family if only he could sell watermelons: "This is the high season and whenever I build my post on the highway for cars to stop and buy, along comes the police and arrests me for causing traffic jams."

The caseworker knew about the situation, but thought there was nothing he could do. For the first meeting of the multiprofessional team, which included the project team—namely, the family therapist, social worker, and project coordinator—several other professionals were also invited. They were the family doctor, who knew all family members from their periodic visits to the local family clinic, teachers of the two school-age boys, a psychiatric social worker who knew the mother from the mental health clinic, and a social worker who was working with girls in distress. It was thought that officials from the "bureaucracy" should also be invited; therefore, a police officer and a representative of the local council were recruited to the team. At the second meeting, the Department of Social Services' community worker who was responsible for the drug program also joined the multiprofessional team.

* * *

Setting up a multiprofessional team is necessary when the family is connected to a variety of agencies and organizations. In the case of the R. family, this included the school system, the clinics, the police, and the Department of Social Services. Another good reason for establishing a multiprofessional team is when the family is stuck, as in our case. The input of other experts in a major and combined effort was needed to implement the objectives of the therapeutic intervention. It is our belief that every human service system should plan according to three objectives: (1) maximization of human potential, (2) prevention of further deterioration of clients' social functioning, and (3) healing of human suffering.

The R. family was suffering for many reasons, and it was clear how this family could be served by all three objectives. Hence, our purpose was to see that the family functioning should not deteriorate further and should be improved as much as possible. It was, therefore, the goal of the MPT to gather the experts, gain more knowledge about family members, share in the knowledge of the participating experts, and set goals that, when reached, would serve to achieve the purpose of the therapy. It was expected that each team member would contribute toward the well-being of the client from the standpoint of the organization that he or she was representing. In the first meetings, the project team presented the family, their recent problems, and what the project would attempt to accomplish. It is worth mentioning that some members of the family in extreme distress may be invited to join the multiprofessional team so that they can be included in, and contribute to, the planned intervention.

The multiprofessional team set several goals. The process took place during two meetings and dealt with the following goals: (1) getting Mr. R. the necessary help to hold a job; (2) arranging for a treatment program for Mrs. R.'s mental health problems; (3) getting A. into an occupational training program; (4) moving B. into a foster home, while working with her and her parents on improving their relationship and helping her to go back to school; (5) working out a suitable study program for the two school-age children, C. and D.; and (6) reevaluating the situation of the younger children, E. and F.

The multiprofessional team set forth a list of tasks to reach the goals that the members had set for themselves. The team also decided to work in pairs on each task. Thus, for example, one task was assigned to the local council representative and the policeman; they were to determine what legal action could be taken to allow Mr. R. to retain his watermelon post in a permitted location. As for Mrs. R., the family doctor and the psychiatric social worker from the mental health clinic were assigned to arrange a rediagnosis of Mrs. R. to establish an appropriate form of treatment. Both the teacher and the family physician indicated that Mrs. R. had been labeled a mental health case, although she was actually functioning well as a mother. The team asked the mental health social worker to coordinate the reevaluation and report to the multiprofessional team at the next meeting.

Another task that was undertaken by the case manager and the community worker was to find a kibbutz A. could join as an outside worker and be trained as a welder, something he had expressed interest in doing.

There was some conflict in regard to the team's goal for B. Some of the team members insisted that she should be placed in a foster family and enrolled in a new school where she could learn a trade. Other members of the team thought she should stay at home and be given more responsibility as the oldest daughter. This would help her mother and improve Mr. R.'s perception of her. It was finally decided that, for the time being, it would be best for B. to leave home. In preparation for such a move, the case manager was asked to look for a foster family and a trade school in another city.

A plan was also drawn up to help C. and D. Several tasks were suggested and agreed upon. The social worker found a Big Brother for the boys. The teachers undertook monitoring the children's difficulties and reporting to the group for further planning.

Finally, it was agreed that a housekeeper should be placed with the family, four hours a day, to help with the young ones, E. and F. The case manager was asked to investigate whether the grandparents would be able to help with the children.

The roles set up for each multiprofessional team member designate specific and well-defined responsibilities to facilitate the execution of the tasks set by the multiprofessional team. This sets the stage for the real challenge for multiprofessional teamwork: the intervention. Accomplishing the assigned tasks leads to achieving the set goals, and once these goals are reached, the solving of problems may begin to take place.

At the following meetings of the multiprofessional team, while the process of intervention took place, the team members received the various reports and were able to make some progress toward their goals. For example, the policeman and council worker reported that Mr. R. would be given a designated location and a permit for the summer season to operate his watermelon post. The team decided that one long-term goal would be to find a permanent location in the new market, to be opened in the coming year. This was in line with Mr. R.'s basic request to find a more secure job. It was suggested that the case manager should help Mr. R. to become better organized in his job search and encourage him to join group therapy to work on controlling his violence.

It was determined that all multiprofessional team members had accomplished their tasks. At that point, another issue was raised for discussion, namely, the R. family debts. The team needed the services of a lawyer to petition the court to combine some of Mr. R.'s debts and spread the payments over a period of time so as to avoid a trial and the likelihood of incarceration. This task was accomplished, as planned, with the lawyer agreeing to become a member of the multiprofessional team.

Most important for the multiprofessional team leader is to follow up on and coordinate the work done by both the team and the caseworkers. Evaluation continues at all stages and steps of the process and is an integral part of the whole process. The multiprofessional team can always start from the beginning, developing new goals and tasks along the way. The multiprofessional team can be expanded by introducing new professionals who might contribute new perspectives and suggest other directions. It is advisable to begin with a small multiprofessional team, adding new members as needed along the way.

In evaluating this case a year later, we were told of the ups and downs of the R. family. The case manager reassessed the efforts invested in the R. family and the progress made: Mr. R. now has his own stall in the market; Mrs. R. functions much better after being reassured by the psychiatrist and the family doctor that she can function with a minimum of medication and only occasional visits to the mental health clinic; the older boy is now in jail for his drug-related activities, but his father maintains contact with him and they discuss future rehabilitation plans; the younger children have improved tremendously and participate in several enrichment programs offered in the community; B. still resides with her foster family, but her relationship with her parents has improved, and she is doing well in school.

These steps taken with the R. family demonstrate what can be accomplished in terms of intervention beyond the therapeutic room. In our project, we used multiprofessional teamwork in order to explore its effectiveness as a working method with FED. In all the cases in which we introduced this method, we found it to be helpful in improving both the family's and the therapeutic team's functioning. We further found that working with a multiprofessional team had helped change some of the team members' negative attitudes toward FED (those who had had previous contact with the family). This affected the different agencies to which they belonged, by spreading positive behavior within the community.

Chapter 8

The L. Family: A Case Study

In this chapter, we will present a description of the therapeutic intervention with the L.s,* one of the families that took part in the project. When the intervention was implemented, the L. family included twelve people: two parents, Mr. and Mrs. L., and their ten children. However, we were told that there had been an older son born with severe physical abnormalities who had died at the age of three (see Figure 8.1).

Mr. L. was born in Morocco and immigrated to Israel, together with his parents, in the early 1960s, at the age of twenty. This move was perceived as a painful and difficult time for both his parents and himself. At the present time, he is recognized as a chronic alcoholic and receives financial support from National Security. In addition, he is working as a gardener in a regional rehabilitation center.

Mrs. L. was born in Morocco and immigrated to Israel as a teenager, together with her parents, in the early 1960s. She comes from a religious background, which is expressed by the many mystical beliefs that she uses to overcome her extreme anxiety. Mrs. L. was hospitalized a few times in a psychiatric department, usually soon after giving birth. She also has some hearing difficulties. As a mother, she takes good physical care of the children and her home.

THE L.s AS A COUPLE AND AS PARENTS

Mr. and Mrs. L. met when Mrs. L. came to visit her cousin who lived close to Mr. L.'s family. Mr. L. fell in love with Mrs. L. and

*For ethical reasons, some of the details about the L. family have been changed, although the therapeutic process is described in full.

FIGURE 8.1. The L. Family

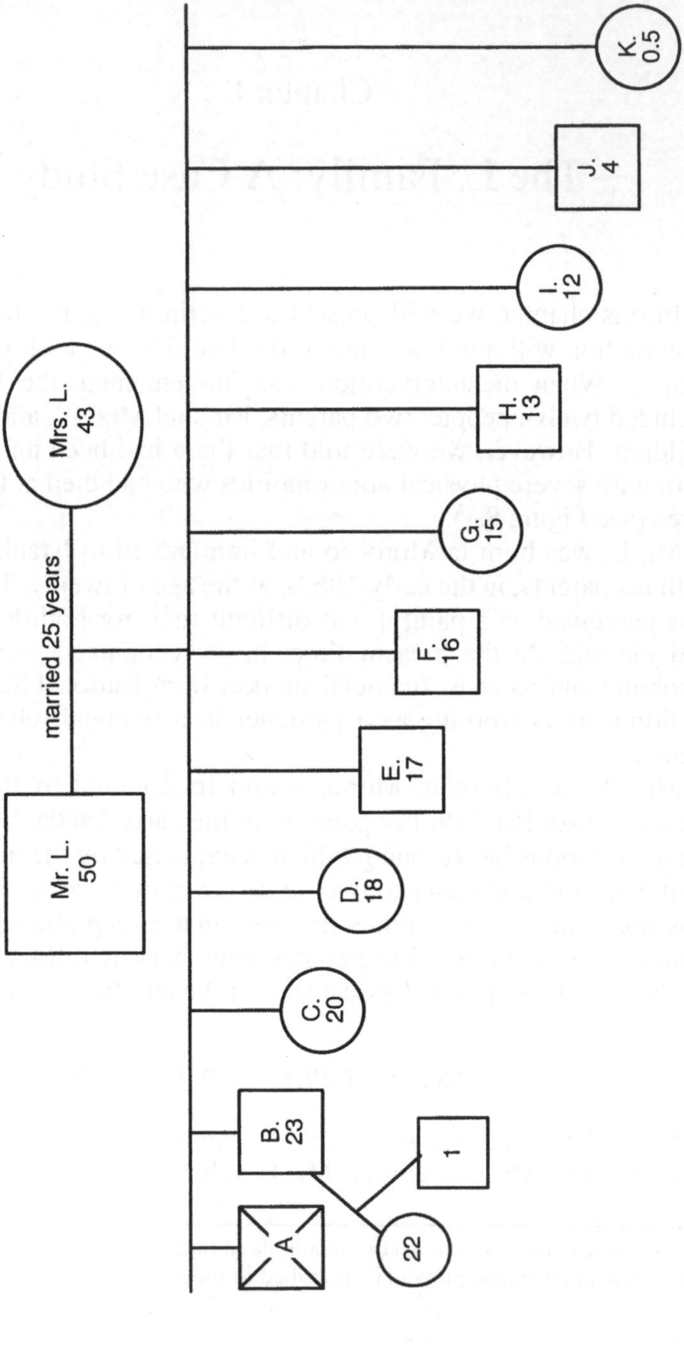

put a lot of pressure on her to marry him. When she refused, he went to her town, which was in another part of the country, and threatened her and her parents that if she did not marry him, he would commit suicide. This emotional threat, issued in the presence of religious people with many mystical beliefs, worked. It was perceived as a sign for "possible death," and Mrs. L. was forced by her father to marry Mr. L. Because of her cultural background, she could not disobey her father's order; thus, she married Mr. L. and moved away to his town.

It is important to note the strong correlation that is usually found between immigration and families in extreme distress. In many cases, the original cultural background, which is usually a traditional one, is disrupted when interacting with the new culture, particularly a Western one. In many families, this causes conflicts between parents and children, sometimes even total disorganization. It seems that the L. family kept its original culture within the Israeli Western society, which might partially account for the members' ability to maintain the family framework in spite of all their difficulties.

Although Mr. L. was supportive, warm, and nurturing toward his wife, he could not relieve her suffering caused by living in close proximity to his side of the family. Mrs. L. was the target of verbal and physical violence by Mr. L.'s brothers. This stopped after the L.s' son was born and they moved to their own apartment. However, memories of this period colored their entire life. Mrs. L. perceived her forced marriage as "bad luck," which was reinforced by her being perceived as a "black sheep" by her husband's family, from whom Mr. L. had not really separated himself. The fact that their first child was born with physical defects also signified continued "bad luck" for her.

The difficult beginnings of the marriage and parenthood, and the continuing daily stresses, sapped Mr. and Mrs. L.'s strength. Mrs. L. experienced mental breakdowns and Mr. L. began drinking. Consequently, some of the children were raised in foster homes and institutions and felt obliged to take on parental roles whenever they returned home. Mr. and Mrs. L. considered it their failure as parents that their children were raised and educated in institutions, but projected their pain and anger on the Department of Social Services as being responsible for taking some of the children from their home.

THE L. FAMILY CHILDREN

A. was born with a major physical defect. When he was about one year old, he was sent to a special institution, where he died two years later. This tragic episode was never fully worked out by the family and is still perceived as the "bad luck" resulting from their forced marriage.

B. is twenty-three, married, and has a son. He lives close to his parents and tries to be helpful. However, both Mr. and Mrs. L. have tried to prevent him from being involved in family difficulties so that "he can keep his marriage." This was perceived by the therapeutic team as a sign of strength on Mr. and Mrs. L.'s part.

C. is twenty years old and serves in the "National Service."* She is close to both her parents and is very helpful, but quiet and introverted. C. was raised in foster families and institutions.

D. is eighteen and is also serving in the "National Service." She was raised at home and moved to a boarding school at age fifteen. She is perceived as the "good girl" who takes care of her mother and the younger children. D. sees herself as a parental figure. Mrs. L. perceives D.'s emerging independence as desertion, but D. is often called upon to come home during small crises, mostly connected to Mrs. L.'s anxiety.

E. is seventeen, was raised in foster homes and institutions, and attends boarding school. He is very quiet and introverted and hardly ever fights for what he wants. Mr. and Mrs. L. threaten to take him back home and not let him graduate if his younger sister "will be sent away to a boarding school."

F. is sixteen, was raised in a foster home, attends boarding school, and is considered to be a good student.

G. is fifteen, lives at home, and goes to a religious school. She complains about the atmosphere at home, the constant fights between her parents and between her and her mother. Her wish to go to a boarding school is strongly supported by the school staff.

H. is thirteen and attends a technical trade boarding school.

---

*Since the family is religious, the girls do not serve in the military, as required in Israel, but instead do one to two years of community service (e.g., in hospitals, schools, or community centers).

I. is twelve and lives with Mr. L.'s sister. She was taken to live with her aunt when she was very young, during one of Mrs. L.'s psychiatric hospitalization periods. I. adjusted very well to her aunt's family, but is conflicted by her mother's anger toward her aunt. Many of the arguments between Mr. and Mrs. L. revolve around this issue.

J. is four years old and attends kindergarten. The teacher reported on his inability to concentrate and his poor verbal skills and has described him as underprivileged because of his poor home environment.

K. is six months old and is well cared for. She seems to be a relaxed baby.

As can be seen, the fact that many of the children are either in foster homes or in educational institutions makes it almost impossible for the family to define its boundaries. This creates anxieties that are the source of many conflicts and crises at home. It also maintains a constant feeling of "bad luck," which seems to have accompanied the family since its inception. In addition to these problems, the family must cope with perpetual financial strain.

The reasons for suggesting therapy to the family, as described by the social worker,* were as follows: (1) G.'s wish to leave home, in addition to her showing signs of suicidal thoughts, was perceived as another threat for the parents, with the potential of destroying the temporary homeostasis reached by the family in regard to raising the children. (2) Mr. L. increased his drinking, became more violent, and started missing work days, which put an additional burden on the family and further exacerbated their financial difficulties. (3) Because of a death in Mr. L.'s sister's family, who had provided a foster home for I., Mrs. L. again began criticizing both Mr. L. and his sister, as well as their daughter I., thus causing conflicts at home and adding to the instability, disorganization, and anxiety.

It was clear that the L. family had the desire to meet the challenge of maintaining the family structure, including raising and educating the children. However, Mr. and Mrs. L. hesitated to join the project because they were afraid that there was a hidden agenda to convince them to let G. leave home.

---

*As described in Chapter 3, the social worker was a member of the therapeutic team, taking on the role of case manager.

THERAPY SESSIONS

The First Session

The entire family, except B., attended the meeting. The therapeutic team supported the family's ability to organize and be at home together for the session. The team began by trying to join the family. This was found to be a very difficult process. While Mr. L. tried to present all the family members to the team, not letting them introduce themselves, he was interrupted by his wife and the younger children. It was clear from the very first minutes of the session that each member of the family was fighting for space within the chaos of the family. After about twenty minutes of trying to join the family, the family therapist understood that without creating some boundaries within the session, she would not be able to join the family. She decided to use two playing cards, one green and one red, made to look like traffic lights; she suggested to family members that the person who wished to talk would hold the green sign and the rest of the family would hold the red sign, remaining silent and listening. These boundaries made it possible to continue the meeting and to find out what the family members hoped to accomplish in the course of the meetings.

It was clear that all of the children suffered from the constant conflicts and fights between the parents; yet all of them supported the mother, who viewed her husband's drinking as the source of the conflicts. It was obvious that the children, especially the daughters, F., D., and G., were involved in these fights, trying to calm their parents and often acting as "judges." Thus, it was easy to see that Mr. L. often felt very lonely when his wife and daughters formed a coalition against him, blaming him for being drunk. This sense of loneliness increased when Mrs. L., along with most of the children, blamed him for the fact that I. was being raised by his sister. While listening to the family story, the family therapist relabeled and redefined some parts of it, as follows:

> **FT:** There are many ways to understand things, but when I see both of you and your children, I have the feeling that you

really care for each one of them. You, Mr. L., help your wife whenever she asks for it, you give her your salary and the National Security support . . . but I see that your wife also cares a great deal for you. She does not want you to drink because it damages your health . . . and both of you care for the children and want to raise them in the best possible way; therefore, you also fight about this issue . . . in fact, most of the fights are about caring, but since it is done by fighting, no one can feel that the other really cares . . .

Although the family members accepted this redefinition, it seemed that they were overwhelmed and could not fully use it to stop the fighting. Mr. and Mrs. L. continued to raise issues concerning Mr. L.'s drinking problem and the fact that Mrs. L. did not recognize Mr. L.'s efforts to help her. At this point, the family therapist, together with the rest of the therapeutic team, tried to challenge the fighting:

FT: Y. [Turning to the case manager], I need your help. It seems to me that there is something about the fights that arouses strong feelings in the couple. I do not know what it is exactly, but it seems to me that there are some codes. It is like a game. For example, Mrs. L. knows that whenever she talks about her husband's drinking, it will end in a fight.

CM: Yes. I agree with you. I was thinking that if Mr. and Mrs. L. did not fight, they would be bored.

FT: [To the children] Do you know how many years your parents have been married?

C.: Yes, twenty-five years.

FT: Twenty-five years and still fighting, but still together? It seems that there is something in these fights that is not like regular fights and we have to find out what it is. But, meanwhile, I would like you to think about something. Whenever you witness your parents fighting and you feel like intervening or calming your parents, or are asked to do so, remember that there is an unknown reason for these fights that has accompanied your parents for twenty-five years. Therefore, it is better that you do not intervene. Just say to one another and to your parents, "We do not interfere or get between you."

With this challenge, the team ended the session. It was clear that there were two issues that bothered the family: the first was the constant fighting between the spouses, which also involved the children, and the second was related to parental issues, especially concerning feelings of failure experienced by the parents. These feelings were primarily focused on G., who wanted to leave home, and I., who had adjusted very well to her foster family but was conflicted by her mother's strong desire for her to return home. A specific agreement was reached regarding attendance for the next meeting. Since it was not possible for E., F., and H. to miss two days at the boarding school to attend the meeting, the team asked them whether it would be possible for them to join a meeting after several weeks, as it was very important for evaluating events occurring in the family. The three boys agreed, and the family asked C., D., G., and I. to join the next meeting. It appeared that the daughters were either more enmeshed in their parents' problems or were the focus of those problems, as with G. and I.

In sum, the first session allowed the initial joining with the family. By creating some boundaries, the family members were able to express their wishes and their pain. After challenging the constant fighting by giving a great deal of support and by relabeling fighting as caring, some of the anxiety was relieved and the family felt encouraged about the prospects of entering therapy.

The Second Session

A week later, when the team arrived, they found Mr. L. drunk and sleeping in his bed, together with his son J. The bed smelled because Mr. L. had thrown up in it and his son had also wet it. Next to the bed was a plate with food, part of which was on the floor, as if he had tried to eat it. While talking with Mrs. L., the team found out that shortly before they had arrived, she and her husband had had a fight, which could be heard in the street—G. had overheard it on her way home from school and now looked very frightened. When the team asked whether it was possible to talk with Mr. L., both Mrs. L. and G. answered that he would probably sleep until the next day. To avoid entering into a coalition with Mrs. L., the team decided to postpone the meeting and use the time for discussion with G. When Mr. L. realized that the team was talking with G., he got up and began a new fight, trying to prevent a connection between the team and G.

The family therapist suggested at that point to divide the session into two parts. During the first part, she and the project director would meet with Mr. and Mrs. L., while the case manager met with G., and during the second part, they would sit together and share the main issues raised in each of the two discussions.

In the discussion with Mr. and Mrs. L., the family therapist found out that Mr. L.'s sister, who had raised I., advised him to quit their participation in the project, since its main goal was to facilitate G.'s leaving home. (It was assumed that the sister, who had raised I. since she was six months old, was afraid that, as a result of the project, I. might return home.) The discussion with his sister increased Mr. L.'s anxiety. Added to this was a visit, together with the baby, K., to Child Health Services, where they were told that the baby needed to be fed only once every four hours, not more. Both Mr. and Mrs. L perceived this as criticism and began to doubt their ability to function as parents. During the entire discussion, both spouses were very anxious, and most of the messages given were meant to reassure them that they were good parents.

In the discussion with G., it was clear that she wanted to leave home, since she could no longer function as the mediator between her parents. She felt that she had not succeeded in this role as well as her older sister D. She also complained that her parents were always comparing her to her sister. The team tried to define her role as a daughter and to acknowledge and support her desire to stay out of her parents' fights. It was decided that, for the time being, she could call the case manager whenever she felt that she was being forced to do things that were inappropriate to the role of a child; the case manager, who had the necessary skills, would mediate between the parents.

Since all of the family members were very anxious following the recent developments, the family therapist decided to use a technique often used by the Milan School at the end of a session, in which a message is given to the family.

FT: To G. and to the therapeutic team] I would like to tell you, G., what I have heard from Mr. and Mrs. L. This family has undergone many difficulties, and they have done it together. When Mrs. L. was hospitalized, Mr. L. took wonderful care of her, like a queen! Besides going with her to the hospital, he went with her to get the Rabbi's blessing. Both of them were afraid and needed a lot of help. Mr. L. helped Mrs. L., who was sick, and Mr. L.'s sister helped him by taking care of the children. Today, Mr. L. feels obligated and loyal to his sister and has become anxious since she advised him to quit the treatment. Yesterday, both Mr. and Mrs. L. became afraid, after visiting the physician, that their baby would be taken away from them. The doctor just suggested that K. should be fed only once every four hours, and, you know, sometimes it is once every four hours, and sometimes every two to three hours. You are the parents, and you know what your baby needs. You have a wonderful baby, and you take very good care of her, but you are so afraid and anxious that the difficult days will return and that Mrs. L. will not be able to take care of the children that every suggestion by a doctor or every bit of advice from a relative becomes a threat. . . . You are even afraid to think about the love you feel toward each other, as Mrs. L. told me today, "Do you think that we would have so many children if we were not in love?" The fights are also a result of the fear.

Mr. L.: Yes, we should not be so afraid.

FT: Let's hear from Y. [the CM] about what happened in her discussion with G.

CM: What we have found out is that you, as parents, care very much for your children and that G., as your daughter, loves and cares very much for both of you and for her brothers and sisters. Yes, you really are a family with a lot of love and caring, but, like yourselves, G. expresses some fears and pain. She wants you to show her that you love and care for her, to hug her, to talk to her, to tell her directly that you love her, and to stop comparing her with D. all the time—

Mrs. L: [Interrupting] Yes, sometimes I take out my anger on her, and it is not her fault.

FT: What you have just said is very important, and I suggest that you talk about it with G. after the meeting. Now let's continue to listen to Y. [Creating focus and boundaries]

CM: There are other things that are important to children as they become teenagers, among which is their peer group. It is essential for children at G.'s age to do things for themselves and not only for the family, such as joining a youth movement. This is very important to G.

Mr. L: But I am afraid to let her go.

FT: Yes, it is very difficult and very frightening to be a teenager's father. Suddenly, children need to do their own thing, and the parents get worried. At the same time, they are happy to see their children growing up, but sad that they are beginning to separate and build their own lives.

Mr. L.: Yes, I am afraid, and I worry about G.

FT: Let's talk about the fear and the worries in our next session. [To the CM in front of the family] Y., please meet with Mr. L.'s sister during the week and try to explain to her that we are on the family's side, not against them. It is important that Mr. L., who is so loyal to his sister, take part in the meeting.

During the second session, it was possible to continue in the direction taken during the first meeting and to explore the nature of the fights. One reason for the fights was Mr. and Mrs. L.'s lack of self-confidence as parents. There was a great deal of reassuring and joining with their fears, in addition to relabeling the fighting as care and love. Included also was the task of joining with the extended family, namely, Mr. L.'s sister, who is enmeshed with the nuclear family. After extensive joining, aimed at creating boundaries, the team began to create some space for G. Since it was clear that the family was still hesitant about joining therapy, the team just set the date for the following meeting, without specifying who should take part in it.

The Third and Fourth Sessions

When the team arrived for the third session, they found that only Mr. and Mrs. L. and D. were present. C. could not come, G., I., and J. were still in school, and K. was sleeping. The meeting began with the team's attempt to rejoin the family. This was very important, since a former social worker for the family had meanwhile intervened in the process and increased Mr. L.'s suspicions. The former social worker had helped Mr. L. while Mrs. L. was sick, and Mr. L. had trusted him very much. During the week, Mr. L. visited the social worker and told him about the project, describing his fears. The social worker, who was working in another agency at the time, suggested that he join one of the sessions to "find out what was going on and advise Mr. L. whether or not to continue with the project." It was clear that Mr. L. was still very anxious, and he indicated that his wife also feared more children being taken away from them. The team suggested that they call the former social worker to tell him about the project, and Mr. L. accepted the suggestion. By doing so, the boundaries of the therapeutic team were redefined. It seemed that the CM's meeting with Mr. L. during the week, which his sister did not attend, was not effective enough in reducing his level of anxiety and feeling overwhelmed; hence, Mr. L. went back to a familiar figure, that of his former social worker.

During the week, the CM visited Child Health Services to find out what had been said to family members that increased their anxiety in the previous session. She explained the intense fears under which the parents lived and requested that the staff be especially careful whenever suggesting something to the family that might cause conflict and affect the overall atmosphere at home. The staff at Child Health Services reported that J. was found to be well-developed and very well cared for by his parents. The CM reported this discussion to the family, focusing on the fact that not only the team but also the staff at Child Health Services recognized their positive functioning as parents.

While listening to this, Mr. L. raised the issue of I. staying with his sister. Bringing up this issue instigated a fight involving Mr. L.,

Mrs. L., and D., but it was not clear whether they really opposed one another. The FT created boundaries by once again using the green and red signs and asking everyone to express his or her point of view.

It was the first time that Mr. L. explained what had happened when his wife had been sick, describing how his sister had helped him and his subsequent loyalty to her. However, he said that he could no longer endure his wife's yelling at him because of his daughter and that he would bring her back home if necessary.

Mrs. L. expressed a great deal of anger toward her sister-in-law for taking her daughter away. She criticized the way in which I. was being educated and raised by the aunt. Mrs. L. became extremely angry when talking about I. joining the mourning ceremonies for the aunt's husband: "According to Jewish tradition, only the wife, their children, the brothers and sisters should sit shivah, a Jewish mourning observance which lasts for seven days and includes certain rituals. I. was not his child—she has a mother and a father. . . . I sent my husband to bring her home, but he did not go. . . . Now it's bad luck and she won't be able to return home for three months."

At this point, C. entered the discussion, indicating that the "three months" is a superstition that does not have anything to do with the Jewish religion. The FT used this opposing view between the mother and the daughter and said, "Your mother is talking about time. She has had a long and painful life experience and knows that sometimes things need time to heal."

This comment changed the direction of the discussion, when Mrs. L. agreed with the FT and said that she still remembered A., their oldest son, who died when he was three years old. Mrs. L. began to tell the story of A. It was the first time that the L.s had spoken about it in detail, in the presence of others, namely, their daughter and the team. The team expressed interest and empathized with their pain. Mrs. L. brought out some pictures of A. At the beginning, she concentrated on the details, with Mr. L. often helping her or adding some details. When the FT focused on feelings, both Mr. and Mrs. L. joined with her and expressed their feelings. When the L.s finished telling their story, the FT connected it with the beginning of the session: "You have had a terrible experience, loss, pain, and sadness. . . . It is the most difficult thing to lose a child, to find that something is not right and to have to move him from one place to another, from one doctor to another, as if he were a package."

Mrs. L.: Yes, and a child is not a package; things have to be done slowly.

FT: Yes, you are right, especially when losing someone.

Mrs. L.: Yes.

FT: At the beginning of the session, you demanded that I. return home. I think that this cannot be done immediately; she is a child, not a package.

Mrs. L.: Yes, not right away, slowly.

Mr. L.: After the shivah, I will tell her to come home and she will decide whether she wants to come or not.

FT: This is too quick; as your wife said, it should be done very slowly, very carefully. Mrs. L., can you explain it to your husband? [Mrs. L. did]

FT: What do you think about meeting with Mr. L.'s sister and talking about your feelings for I.?

Mrs. L.: Yes, I agree.

Mr. L.: We will invite her to the next meeting.

Mrs. L.: No, she cannot enter this house. It is bad luck—her husband died; we will go to her house.

FT: Let us know where we are going to meet next week. The CM will meet separately with G., just like last week.

Mr. L.: Why? She told me that you said she could go to boarding school.

CM: Nothing like that was said. I will meet with G. because, as we said last week, children her age have to do things for themselves.

D.: G. told me that she took the entry exams for the boarding school in Kfar-Pinnes* and was accepted.

FT: If she was accepted to Kfar-Pinnes, it means that you have a very talented daughter. However, nothing was said about leaving home.

The following week, the L.s met with Mr. L.'s sister, the aunt and foster mother of I., at her house, together with the team. During this meeting, the aunt described her feelings toward I. and I. described her own feelings toward her parents and her aunt. She asked her parents to accept her wish to stay with the aunt without ignoring her. The parents, who for the first time listened to the aunt and to their daughter, tended to agree. This was supported by the FT who said, "Sometimes good parents give up their own wishes for their children, and I see that you are ready to do it. You understand that it is important for your daughter, although very difficult for you." The parents accepted I.'s request, and the issue did not come up again in such an intensive way until the end of the therapeutic process.

It seems that the parents' ability to tell the narratives of the family in the presence of witnesses and the acknowledgment and support they received helped them in letting I. separate without having to cut off from the family completely. It also created boundaries between the L.s, who were defined as "the family," and Mr. L.'s sister, who was defined as the "foster family." These boundaries reduced the invisible loyalty of Mr. L. toward his sister, which was the source of many fights between Mr. and Mrs. L.

The Fifth Session

The fifth session began late since the family went shopping and did not organize the time well. The session took place during winter vacation. Boys E., F., and H. were at home, providing a good opportunity to involve them in the therapeutic process. C. and D. were busy with National Service, and G. went to visit relatives in another town. When talking with the boys, it was clear that all of them enjoyed coming home from their boarding schools. The team,

---

*A very prestigious religious boarding school.

therefore, used the meetings to increase the parents' self-confidence by listening to the boys' stories and emphasizing points where the children described positive experiences with the parents:

> **E.:** I like to come home very much. . . . No matter when I come—it can be in the middle of the night—Mom will get up and prepare something to eat. She is great.
>
> **FT:** Mrs. L., do you hear what your son is saying about you, that you are a caring mother?
>
> **Mrs. L.:** [Smiling] Yes, they are my life.
>
> **FT:** And what about Dad?
>
> **E.:** When he drinks, no one can talk to him, but when he is sober, there is no one like him. No one.
>
> **FT:** No one like your father! Do you hear that, Mr. L.? . . . I wonder, since you and F. were at home when your mother got sick, do you remember how Dad took care of you?
>
> **F.:** Yes, of course. It was very difficult because we were young and he had to run between us and the hospital.
>
> **E.:** Until he could not do it anymore and we went to foster families. We always like to come home; the only things that bother us are the fights and Dad's drinking.
>
> **FT:** You were not here during all the meetings, but we found out that beyond the fights, your parents really love each other. You could see how your Dad took care of your mother when she was sick and how he took care of you.

The FT tried to tip the balance in the situation to create a place for the father beyond his drinking problems. The fact that the boys were at home and that Mr. L. was not surrounded only by females provided a good opportunity to acknowledge him. It was obvious that the family had accepted that the boys were in boarding school or in foster homes, but that they could not accept the same for the daughters. When the FT made this observation, Mrs. L. raised the issue with G.: "Yes, they are boys, and G. should help at home." She continued to complain about G., voicing most of the usual objections about a teenager. When the project director (PD) heard them, she joined the discussion:

> **PD:** You know, Mrs. L., I am not so old, only about nine or ten years older than G., and I remember behaving just like G. toward my mother. I wanted to show my mother that I was a grown-up and smarter than her, but I really loved her and was ashamed to show her how I felt.
>
> **Mrs. L.:** Yes, yes.
>
> **CM:** You know, I met G. this week, just after your fight when you hit her. G. told me that in spite of all the fighting, she loves you. I am thinking now that it would be a good idea to meet just with the two of you, mother and daughter.
>
> **Mrs. L.:** Okay, but what about the boarding school? The counselor from the school wants her to come to the school.
>
> **FT:** I think it is a wonderful idea that you, Mrs. L., G., and the CM meet during the week. We will try to arrange a meeting with the school counselor. I am sure that we can find a way for both you and G. to enjoy each other.

This meeting continued to direct the intervention toward increasing the parents' confidence, thereby helping them to take on more parental roles and freeing the children from such obligations. After the fifth session, the parents still needed considerable reinforcement, but they had begun to trust the team.

The Sixth Session

After the fifth session, the CM contacted the school and suggested arranging a joint meeting with the L. family. The counselor agreed, but she asked to postpone it for a week due to prior commitments. The CM contacted the L.s and reminded them about the upcoming meeting, telling them that it would be without the school counselor. When the team arrived at the L.s' residence, they found that only Mrs. L. was at home, appearing disorganized and not knowing where

Mr. L. was to be found. To avoid any possible coalition with Mrs. L., or any indication that might point to Mr. L. as "being an outsider," the family therapist suggested that they wait outside the apartment for fifteen minutes. If Mr. L. did not show up, they would postpone the meeting until the following week. This arrangement helped Mrs. L. to organize her thoughts. She thanked the team members and returned to look after her baby, who had started crying.

Mr. L. arrived while the team was waiting outside the apartment. He too seemed disorganized. The FT suggested that the couple take a few minutes, have some coffee together, and get organized. The meeting was started twenty minutes later. The ability of the team to contain the disorganization of the couple, instead of judging it, was important for the family, who were used to judgmental attitudes on the part of members of social institutions, such as teachers at the children's schools or health professionals at the clinics.

It was understood by the team members that disorganization and lack of boundaries were part of the family's problems and had to be worked on in therapy rather than expecting the family to instantly change simply because it had agreed to join the project. Such disorganized behavior is often interpreted by professionals as a lack of motivation for change, followed by a negative attitude toward the clients and further exacerbation of the coalition of despair. Regarding such behavior as the target of the treatment, as well as the family's way of defining its daily lifestyle, turns the therapist's criticism into a challenge. Thus, therapy becomes an opportunity rather than a context for control.

Mr. L. prepared coffee for his wife and the team, receiving a great deal of praise for his effort. This helped him to apologize for being late and to explain the reason. He had gone to find out about his salary because of their terrible financial situation, which worried him day and night. The understanding and support he received from the team produced a certain imbalance that seemed to threaten Mrs. L. In fact, it changed the image that she had tried to present of herself as "the good one," while her husband was "the drunk, violent bad guy." As a result, she began criticizing her husband's drinking, his using their money for beer, and his becoming violent when drunk. It appeared that Mrs. L.'s anxiety was going to overwhelm the team and the session, when suddenly Mr. L. spoke to the FT:

Mr. L.: Please ask her what is the reason for this behavior.

FT: [To Mrs. L.] Why don't you tell us? I am sure you have something on your mind, and we are very interested to hear it from you.

Mrs. L.: [Continued to blame, criticize, and yell]

FT: Let's try to make up a rule. There is a banana and an orange here. You, Mr. L., take the banana, which will represent a sign to talk, while you, Mrs. L., take the orange, which will be a sign to listen, and later on you will change.

[Mr. L. tried to speak again, but the recommended signs were not sufficient, and Mrs. L. was still very anxious and overwhelmed.]

FT: [To the CM] Y., this is very difficult for Mrs. L. It seems to bring up painful and frightening memories. I suggest that you sit next to her and help her listen to Mr. L.

[The CM moved close to Mrs. L. and put her hand on Mrs. L.'s shoulder. Mrs. L. smiled and was then able to listen to Mr. L.]

Mr. L. told the story of their family. He described his efforts in helping Mrs. L. when she was sick, the way he went with her from one doctor to another, from one hospital to another. He talked about his despair when he realized that he could not take proper care of Mrs. L. and the children at the same time. He described how he turned to drinking as a way of overcoming his despair. With great sorrow, he expressed his need for acknowledgment and recognition from Mrs. L., which he never received, in spite of his efforts to help her. Mr. L.'s story was listened to with a great deal of interest and acknowledgment by the team, as they learned about his efforts to be a caring husband and father:

FT: You are a wonderful and caring husband. You want so much for your wife and children. You refer to your wife as a queen. Did you notice it [to Mrs. L.]?

Mrs. L.: [Smiling] Yes.

FT: So, when you heard his story, could you feel how he cares for you?

Mrs. L.: Yes, he did all this because he loves me, but I want him to stop drinking because when he is drunk, he is violent. No one can talk with him when he yells, hits, and breaks things.

FT: Yes, Mr. L. was ready to do so many things that he forgot himself when he became an alcoholic. It is very difficult to overcome this.

Mr. L.: I want to stop drinking and go for treatment, but how will she stay here alone with the children and all the household problems? And what about money?

FT: Yes, I agree that neither of you is ready yet for substance control therapy. Proper arrangements will have to be made for this.

Mrs. L.: I want him to stop drinking.

FT: Yes, of course, you care about him and also do not want to suffer from his violence. [The FT continued to talk about setting up clear boundaries, about violence and its being against the law, and about how Mrs. L. had a right to protect herself and the children by calling the police if necessary. She added that they obviously cared for each other and emphasized their painful family history.]

Three issues made up the main theme of this meeting: (1) rejoining with family members and accepting their disorganization rather than criticizing them as being "unmotivated," while challenging them to organize themselves; (2) giving Mr. L. the opportunity to tell his story, acknowledging his pain and caregiving, and thereby creating some imbalance in the "good guy/bad guy" image of the spouses; and (3) creating boundaries by allowing Mr. L. to talk without interruption and by taking a clear stand against Mr. L.'s violent behavior.

The Seventh Session

This session focused on discussions with G.'s counselor and educator and on the possibility of sending her to a very prestigious religious boarding school. The school staff recognized G.'s intellectual potential and the tensions at home that prevented her from concentrating on her studies. The school staff put a great deal of pressure on the therapeutic team to convince, or even force, the family to let G. go to boarding school. The team presented another point of view. Even though they recognized the advantages of studying at the boarding school, they did not see any reason for the use of force, or legal means, to pressure the family. On the contrary, the team was of the opinion that the only way for G. to attend boarding school was by obtaining her parents' blessing; otherwise, she risked guilty feelings and unresolved conflicts with her parents, which would impede her ability to concentrate on her studies.

During the session, the parents received a great deal of support and acknowledgment for the way in which they had raised their children. The counselor and the educator described the way that they remembered the two elder daughters, who were excellent students, but emphasized G.'s special intellectual talents, which, in their opinion, would be expressed much better in boarding school. The family therapist then summarized the counselor's and educator's comments in order to focus the parents and join with the family.

> **FT:** What I have heard from the counselor and the educator was that you are caring parents, which can be seen by looking at your children. However, the teachers see G. as a very special and talented girl and are trying to find the best educational environment for her, where she can use and express all her talents. That is why they recommend this boarding school. What do you think? You are the parents, and you know what is best for your children.

> **Mr. L.:** [Assuming his role as the father, he began expressing his point of view. It appeared that the place he was given in the sixth session had been effective.] C. and D. studied in G.'s school and it was an excellent school for them, so why not for G.? We are always in contact with the school and come to parents' meetings where you can talk to me about G. I do not want her to leave home, and if you do it by force, I will bring F. back home from his boarding school and I. from my sister.

Mrs. L.: If G. leaves home, no one will remain to help me.

[The counselor and educator then entered into conflict with the parents about G.'s role in the family, which escalated the tension in the room.]

FT: First of all, it is important for us to say that no one is going to force you to send G. to the boarding school. You are good parents, and we do not have any reason to force you to do something that you do not wish for your daughter. However, the children are not exchangeable items: it is not "either G. stays home or I will . . ."; we have to think about what is best for each one of them.

It was clear that G. maintained the homeostasis in the family and that, by remaining at home, she reduced her parents' pain over I. being raised by her aunt, also acting as mediator between the parents. It was also clear, as later expressed by the parents, that it was not possible for them to let the girls leave home, either to boarding schools or other institutions, and that it was easier for them to let the boys go. The team recognized this, but did not see a way to work it out at this stage of the treatment. As the meeting proceeded, Mrs. L. was ready to think about the possibility of G. studying at a boarding school, but asked to postpone it for a year. Mr. L. was still threatened by the fact that G. would be taken away by force, with the help of the law. Although the FT repeatedly tried to make it clear that G. would not be taken to boarding school without the parents' permission, Mr. L. was not convinced.

The Eighth and Ninth Sessions

When the team arrived for the eighth session, Mr. L. was in his room, drunk and half asleep. Mrs. L. said that it had been a very difficult week and asked G. to join her and to tell the team about Mr. L.'s behavior. Before G. had a chance to speak, Mr. L. entered the room and began to yell. Mrs. L. talked to him in a soft voice, asking him to go and rest. The team joined her by saying that they were leaving because he needed the rest and would return next week. Mr. L. became angry and violent and said that he wanted to stop therapy. He threw a chair in the direction of his wife. The therapist suggested that everyone leave the apartment, since violence presented danger. Mrs. L., the children, and part of the team left the apartment. The FT tried in vain to calm down Mr. L. Meanwhile, Mrs. L. called the police, and when they arrived, she refused to complain. The police officer advised Mrs. L. to file a complaint so that they could take her husband to the police station for a few hours, where he might rest and sober up, but she refused. She also refused to leave the house for a few hours to keep herself and the children away from the violence. The team became very anxious and was at a loss about what to do. It was the police officer who told the team not to worry because Mrs. L was used to this kind of situation and would know what to do. He added that if Mrs. L. thought there was actual danger, she would not have refused his advice or the team's suggestion to leave home. The FT accepted the police officer's point of view, reinforcing Mrs. L.'s ability to relate to her husband in such a situation. However, the FT repeated the police officer's advice as well as her own. Meanwhile, the police officer entered the apartment and reported that Mr. L. was fast asleep and that the situation seemed safe. Mrs. L. and the children returned to the apartment, and the team scheduled the next meeting with the family.

In the supervisory session between the eighth and ninth meetings, the FT worked on her own fears and the way in which they affected the situation at hand, as well as the entire team. Since the team was still anxious, it was decided to invite Mr. and Mrs. L. to the DSS office for the ninth meeting to do some debriefing and to try to rejoin with Mr. L. It was assumed that the seventh meeting with the school counselor had generated undue strain on the parents, which was expressed by Mr. L.'s heavy drinking about one week after the meeting. The ninth meeting took place in the DSS office. The team members prepared coffee and tea for Mr. and Mrs. L., stating that, this time, they had the opportunity to host the L. family:

FT: I would like to explain why we wanted to have the meeting here. Last week . . .

Mr. L.: I was crazy.

FT: Crazy?

Mr. L: I found out that I owe a great deal of money. I haven't paid my water bills for eight months, and when I went to talk to the manager, he got angry and we had a fight. I told him that I had a big family, that I was sick and could not pay so many bills, but he would not help. Finally, he agreed to split the debt into several installments, and I gave him my bank account number so that the bills can be deducted directly from the account. When I got home, I. came in for just a minute and left. I told her that if she wanted to come home, she was always welcome, but if she did not want to, no one was forcing her.

FT: Who forced I. to come home?

Mr. L.: You spoke to my sister, and she forced her to come home.

FT: Maybe your sister did not understand, and we will have to call her and explain that we did not mean for her to force I. to leave. However, last week, when we came to you . . .

Mr. L.: I was crazy.

FT: You were in pain, which hurt all of us—yourself, your wife, your children, and us [referring to the therapeutic team].

Mr. L.: My pain was the greatest. You told me that G. was going to boarding school. If such a thing happens, the family and the house will be destroyed; I will destroy it . . . [he continues to describe his pain].

FT: It must have been very painful.

Mr. L.: Yes.

FT: It's a pity because we told you very clearly that G. would not go to boarding school without your "blessing" and that no one would force you to send her, but you were still afraid, became depressed, and started drinking. You already know what happened later on. You are a good husband and a good father, and you take very good care of your family, but then you destroyed everything by getting drunk.

Mrs. L.: I want you to stop drinking—it destroys you and us.

Mrs. L. sat quietly while her husband described his pain. This marked a definite change in the couple's communication. Mrs. L. was able to listen to him and to be part of the team's effort in joining with her husband, while not feeling left out. It remained to be seen whether this was a real change, or just a pseudochange, since the content of the discussion focused on "Mr. L.'s problem." The team took this into account when Mrs. L. repeated the request that her husband stop drinking and that the FT intervene:

> **FT:** [To the CM] I wonder what Mrs. L. knows about the treatment for alcohol abuse. It's often a family project. Do you know something about it?
>
> **CM:** I know that the family must be prepared to give a lot of help and support. First of all, the patient will have to be placed in a special institution, located at a distance of about three hours from here, for several months. Some work will have to be done with his wife, and upon his return home, he will need a great deal of support.
>
> **FT:** We have to find out whether Mr. L. and Mrs. L. are ready for it.

This was the first time that the couple communicated about the issue of Mr. L.'s drinking in such an atmosphere. Mrs. L. did not blame her husband, but rather tried to explain the damage caused by his drinking and to convince him to take better care of himself. The team acknowledged the change in communication and supported both spouses. At the end, the FT stated that the alcohol issue needed further work, and since the following session was to be the last one, the family would have to decide if they wanted to continue dealing with the issue together with the CM.

The Tenth Session

The family succeeded in organizing itself in such a way that all the children arrived for the last meeting. The FT began by describing the therapeutic process, while the entire family listened quietly. This was quite different from the first session, when definite boundaries were required to create some order. Next, the therapist requested the parents' permission for the children to present their perspectives about what was happening in the family and asked whether they would be ready to listen to the children. After getting the parents' approval, the therapist asked the children how they saw the current situation in the family and what they expected to happen in the future.

All of the children stated that there seemed to be some changes in the relationship between the parents following treatment. Although there were still fights and conflicts, these now seemed to be less intense. C. and D. indicated that the task of not intervening in their parents' fights, assigned to them at the first meeting, had been very helpful, even though, at the time, it had seemed to be artificial and impossible to implement. Most of the children talked about the feeling of hope that had returned—the hope that their parents would again get along and function as a family. By functioning, they meant that their father would stop drinking and their mother would not be angry all the time. All of the children acknowledged the efforts that the parents had invested in their upbringing and education. G. surprised the family and the team when she announced that she had decided to remain at home and to postpone her studies at the boarding school. She told the team about the significant improvement in her relationship with her mother, which had raised her spirits and stopped her suicidal thoughts. She reassured her family that she had never actually intended to commit suicide, but rather used the threat as a means to force them to send her to boarding school. She then said that she preferred to have the parents' blessing to go to boarding school rather than to go against their wishes. She confirmed that the individual therapy sessions, as well as the joint sessions with her mother, had contributed a great deal to her decision to remain at home for the present time. G., similar to the rest of the children, regarded hope as the main product of the therapeutic process. Mr. and Mrs. L. joined in their children's observations:

> **Mr. L.:** Many things have changed. First of all, my wife does not yell as much . . . when I come home from work, she treats me with respect and I can forgive her yelling and cursing. Because of this, I drink less . . . we can often talk quietly now. . . . I am happy because G. has decided to remain at home.

Mrs. L.: Things have changed. . . . I am not afraid of my husband because he does not beat me anymore. . . . When he does not drink, he helps out with the children. G. is more relaxed now, and last week, I. came to visit several times, not only for a minute. She stayed longer and we talked . . .

From the family members' comments, it was clear that, in addition to their renewed hope, they perceived a change in their ability to listen and to express their thoughts and feelings. The team summarized the therapeutic process by using the metaphor of a garden because Mr. L. worked as a gardener in his rehabilitation program:

FT: You are like a garden that used to be so well looked after. Over the years, some of the plants failed, and in spite of his efforts, the gardener could not succeed in saving them all or in doing all the work that was needed. He was jumping from one plant to another. When he was able to save one, another plant died. Eventually, many of the plants died and the weeds multiplied to the point that it became impossible to tell the flowers from the weeds. Yet, now it seems that all of these efforts were not lost, and some changes have begun to appear. We see flowers blooming again, with clear spaces between the plants. This gives us renewed energy to care for what used to be a beautiful garden with deep roots.

Mr. L: Thank you, you brought us a lot of happiness.

The family continued to work with the CM for another year, all the while consulting with the family therapist. The ability to communicate lasted throughout the year. With the family's support, Mr. L. started his alcohol abuse treatment. G. no longer brought up her wish to leave home, and I. continued to visit the family. There were still occasional fights and conflicts between the spouses, but fewer than before the therapeutic process. Although the family's financial situation did not improve, the family seemed better able to organize its income and expenditures. It seemed that the spirit of hope, brought on during the three months of intensive intervention, permeated the family and had a lasting effect, thus preventing a coalition of despair with the CM.

SUMMARY OF THE THERAPEUTIC INTERVENTION

What has been accomplished by the intervention? Why has it worked? When analyzing the process, it was found that most of the therapeutic techniques used by the team were "preparing techniques," such as joining and rejoining, reassuring, supporting, reframing, and empowering.

Two main themes became the target for intervention. The first theme involved parental perspectives and focused on the parents as good parents who "care for their children and are ready to do anything in order to help them, such as sending them out to foster homes or boarding schools if these would offer them a better education." The second theme involved spousal perspectives and focused on conflicts concerning the drinking and violence and the inability to accomplish the overwhelming load of household chores.

The therapeutic process provided a new experience for the family. For the first time, family members did not feel judged or targeted for change by the social agents, but rather empowered and supported. This was the main accomplishment of the intervention. Due to its painful history with social institutions, the family had to overcome many obstacles, but, fortunately, these were perceived as a challenge for the team to rejoin with family members, rather than to label them as "unmotivated."

Only when a measure of trust was established, did the team use "changing techniques," such as creating direct communication and unbalancing. This gave Mr. L. a place in the family, not only as a drunk and violent man, but as a caring husband and father. The direct communication created some boundaries between the children and the parents and reduced the children's roles as mediators and parental children. All of this helped to reduce the frequency and severity of the family's fights.

We wondered whether a longer, more intensive intervention was needed or whether another series of interventions should have been recommended for a few months later. We were of the opinion that the family needed a break period between interventions in order to experience the changes achieved. We were convinced that ten additional intensive meetings would have served to reinforce what had been accomplished. Unfortunately, as is often the case with welfare policies, lack of funds prevented the project from continuing. However, the hope that was rekindled within the family, as well as the actual change effected, cannot be underestimated. Furthermore, the ability of the CM to rejoin the family from a perspective of hope rather than through maintenance of the coalition of despair affected her relationship with the family and the process of intervention long after the project had ended.

Have all the family's problems been solved? Definitely not. Could family members function without some help from the Department of Social Services? The answer is still no, but their problems appear to be less intense and their coping more effective and free of despair.

Chapter 9

Supervision in the Context of Therapy with Families in Extreme Distress

The goal of supervision in family therapy and in social work is to help therapists and social workers provide useful service to the clients within their agency (Burnham, 1993). However, in practicing supervision, this goal is translated into different modes, with different targets. Some approaches highlight the development of knowledge and skills (Feldman, 1977; Haley, 1976; Kadushin, 1985; Madanes, 1986), whereas other approaches perceive supervision as an empowering process, used mainly in supporting and encouraging supervisors to discover and implement their skills (Anderson, 1988; Arndt, 1955; Elkaim, 1997; Vargus, 1977). In the process of intervention with FED, it seems to us that there are benefits in an integrative approach that makes use of different, yet complementary, goals (Burnham and Harris, 1992; Burnham, 1993; Kaslow, 1986; Munson, 1983).

As indicated in previous chapters that described the techniques utilized in interventions with FED, the complexity of treating this population requires the freedom to use different means, without being committed to a single approach. This is also true for the process of supervision in which the overwhelming range of problems affects therapists and social workers in various ways. They often require actual skills and tools, while at other times they need more in the way of reassurance and assistance. The supervisor thus empowers them to discover a different level of understanding and another way of approaching the family. In this manner, the supervisor who provides ongoing support and encouragement moves between the various roles of teacher, role model, support giver, therapist, and colleague (Sharlin and Chaiklin, 1998).

As teacher, the supervisor offers the theoretical and practical knowledge that is needed at specific points in the intervention.

As role model, the supervisor functions on many levels. In the context of life supervision, this might mean giving direct instructions about what to do. At other times, the supervisory meeting might take the form of a consultation, namely, working with the family under the direction of the supervisor, while the supervisees observe the procedure. The supervisory context creates a relationship in which the supervisees benefit from the freedom to express feelings and thoughts, can discover and relate to positive as well as negative feelings toward the clients, and are able to reach a new understanding of the clients and the intervention process. The supervisees can also utilize this type of dialogue, which is being created during the supervisory process while working with the family, as a means of increasing their potential, to strengthen personal and professional growth.

As a giver of support, the supervisor contains the frustrations and disappointments of the supervisees, without blaming them for entering into such an emotional state. As described in Chapter 3, when reaching a point of frustration during intervention with FED, there is often a sense of hopelessness and helplessness. Accepting this as one aspect of the therapeutic process is part of learning how to cope with despair. Here, the supervisor allows a parallel process to the therapy itself, wherein the feelings of the supervisees are acknowledged and contained by the supervisor, just as clients' feelings are expected to be contained by the therapist (the supervisee) when working with FED.

As therapist, the supervisor helps the supervisees to be aware of the "resonance" emitted during a meeting with a specific family in a specific context (Elkaim, 1997). From the large number and variety of problems that FED bring to the therapeutic situation, some may be associated with the supervisees' own personal and family history. Since the problems presented tend to be extremely severe, the therapist's tone might awaken feelings of anxiety, thus limiting therapeutic capability. It is, therefore, the role of the supervisor to help supervisees discover their own resonance and to differentiate between their personal experience and that of the family, while using this experience to gain a better understanding of the family. It is not the role of the supervisor to be the supervisee's therapist, and the boundaries between supervision and therapy should be clear and maintained. However, the supervisor should touch upon such resonance as is relevant to the supervisees' ability to help their clients, as well as that which is relevant to their own professional growth.

As a colleague, the supervisor creates a situation wherein the supervisees are able to take part in a multilevel dialogue dealing with professional and nonprofessional issues. This allows the supervisees to be critical of their clients and the agencies and to use sarcastic language or jokes. It is an opportunity to share professional experience, without necessarily using it directly as material for supervision. This nonhierarchical situation generates a discussion that enables a "time-out" from the tensions created by working with FED.

Many topics and issues arising in the supervision of family therapists and social workers working with FED are similar to those of regular family therapy supervision. However, five topics seem to be unique and have specific relevancy to the supervision of those working with FED: (1) coping with the coalition of despair (COD) before and during the therapeutic process; (2) coping with the anger of FED toward society that is directed at the therapist or social worker as representatives of society; (3) coping with the family's overwhelmed condition; (4) developing a systematic view rather than an individual perspective focused on the wife/mother; and (5) relating to the entire team. These five topics are interrelated and often overlapping. Therefore, by focusing on one topic, we might also relate to the other topics.

COPING WITH THE COALITION OF DESPAIR BEFORE AND DURING THE THERAPEUTIC PROCESS

As described in Chapter 3, one of the main problems in working with FED is the coalition of despair between FED and the therapists/social workers (Shamai and Sharlin, 1996). This coalition creates feelings of mistrust, hopelessness, and helplessness among therapists involved in the case, similar to those of the family. The profusion of problems and their long history and severity increases the possibility for entering into such a coalition. Therefore, it is essential to prepare the therapist before the therapeutic process begins. It is necessary to train the therapist in identifying clues that may lead them toward despair, to define the clues, and to include them in the supervision. Let us illustrate the case of therapist S.:

> In one of the therapeutic meetings, family therapist S. presented a situation that she, herself, defined as a situation of despair. According to the therapist, the only change that was possible and needed was a change in the family's financial situation. The couple had triplets, less than one year old, who needed a special kind of baby food. In addition, the services of a mother's helper, provided by Social Security, had been discontinued at the end of the year, so the mother had to take care of the three babies on her own. The couple told the team about their inability to provide food and other basic needs for daily living. At the end of the session, the family therapist called the supervisor, sounding desperate and overwhelmed by the family's situation. After telling the story, the family therapist added, "We are talking about very basic needs. What can I tell them about their marital relationship (which was the target of the intervention) after hearing their story? It is completely irrelevant." It seems that the family therapist, together with the entire team, was about to join the family to form a coalition of despair.
>
> The supervisor allowed the therapist to repeat the story of the family several times, while the supervisor listened and showed interest by asking questions and reassuring the therapist that the situation was indeed difficult and complicated. Moreover, the supervisor validated the therapist's assessment that without first attending to the family's basic needs, the psychological problems could not be addressed. Afterward, the supervisor pointed out to the therapist the dangers of joining the family's despair and consequently being rendered powerless to help its members. This was a clear turning point at which the family therapist refocused on the problem of finances and began to look for ways to solve the problem and improve the family's condition. Listening and observing the therapist's attempts to solve the family's problems, the supervisor reassured the supervisee that she appreciated her ability to join with family members and

empathize with them, as a result of which she was able to find helpful solutions for them.

In the supervisory session that took place two days later, the therapist presented a different situation. She said that the family had experienced such situations before and survived; therefore, she decided to use the present crisis to help the family reorganize to increase its income. For example, she urged the husband to renegotiate his salary, which was below minimum wage, and encouraged the mother to arrange help from the extended family for a few hours every day. The therapist described how it became possible to integrate the therapeutic goal, as defined by the family, with the current crisis.

At that point, the supervisor asked the therapist what it was in the family's "basic needs" and "financial security" that made her so anxious about the family. Also, what was her own personal resonance that caught her in the despair and later helped her to overcome it, turning it instead into a challenge? The therapist made the connection between the family's financial situation and her own conceptions, but added that she was not aware of what triggered the change in her attitude toward the family. However, she indicated that being able to call the supervisor when she needed to discuss the case was very important to her. The comment made by the supervisor about her ability to join the family at such a deep level created an inner dialogue for the therapist. The supervisee appreciated the comment and the endorsement of her clinical skills, but also began to wonder whether she had overidentified with the family's problems. In consideration of the supervisor's comments about her attempts to solve the family's problems, she began separating herself from the family and from the sensation of being overwhelmed by these problems; she was therefore able to use her therapeutic skills more effectively. Working on the supervisee's resonance, which seemed to have evolved from her own family of origin (Elkaim, 1997), provided further understanding and helped her to better relate to the family and to other FED, without entering into a coalition of despair in similar situations.

This example illustrates how easy it is to create a coalition of despair with families in extreme distress. In this situation, the supervisory process prevented further deterioration, and, thus, only three components of the coalition of despair were expressed, namely disorganization and lack of boundaries, a concrete way of thinking, and hopelessness and helplessness. The severe financial situation overwhelmed the therapist, and her overidentification with the family blurred the boundaries between herself and the family, allowing her to become hopeless and helpless along with family members. This was expressed by her concrete way of thinking, which blocked her from being open to other alternatives for change. Thanks to the supervisory process, the coalition was thwarted on its way to becoming a full-blown, change-buffering situation.

COPING WITH THE ANGER OF FED TOWARD SOCIETY THAT IS DIRECTED AT THE THERAPIST OR SOCIAL WORKER AS REPRESENTATIVES OF SOCIETY

Most FED feel a great deal of anger toward society, blaming it for creating and maintaining the condition that is responsible for their despair. Although the anger and the blaming of society is sometimes reality based, there are many situations in which this blaming is used as a way to project one's responsibility away from oneself. This anger is usually directed toward those who are perceived as representatives of society. Thus, social workers and other mental health professionals who work in public services are perceived as a "social institute" rather than as human beings who are trying to provide assistance, consequently becoming a target for FED's aggression.

When anger and blame are projected toward social workers and mental health professionals, a very complicated interactive system is created. Through the process of projective identification, the professionals enter the role of "social institute" and feel blamed by their clients. Feeling accused and blamed prevents their effective use of therapeutic skills. These professionals often try to reduce the blame through overidentification with society and by blaming the families for not taking responsibility for their own lives. Furthermore, identification with society does not challenge FED to take on more responsibility; on the contrary, it increases the anger of FED toward the therapists and toward society. Furthermore, it strengthens this somewhat unrealistic unification between mental health professionals and society. In addition, overidentification with the client against society at large may lead to a coalition of despair.

In the process of supervision, it is important to help therapists to break away from this interactive loop by differentiating between themselves, as professionals and human beings, and society, as represented by its social institutions. When such a differentiation is clarified, the therapists are able to be more empathic about the anger and the blame and are thus better able to work through these feelings with the family. The main questions underlying the topic of supervision are "To whom does the anger belong?" and "Who takes responsibility for it?" To proceed with the therapeutic process, family therapists must be able to give negative answers to both questions, namely, that the anger does not belong to them, but to FED and/or society, and that these two, not the therapists, are responsible for it. The role of the family therapists and social workers is to help the family and society to deal with the anger by providing intervention as well as by recommending appropriate social services to the FED population. Let us illustrate this through the case of the SA. family:

> As the family therapist described the therapeutic sessions, it became clear that every session began with the family members' expressions of anger toward society, especially toward the Department of Social Services, without taking any responsibility for creating and maintaining their enormous amount of problems. Mr. SA. claimed that although the social workers tried to rehabilitate him, "it was not good enough." He was still deeply in debt, but "the social workers are not doing enough to help me get out of debt." The endless complaints and anger affected the family therapist, and she became angry at the family, feeling that she was "tired" of them and did not want to meet with them any longer. She raised this issue at the supervisory meeting.
>
> The supervisor first tried to define the nature of Mr. SA.'s anger and to determine toward whom it was directed. It was

> made clear to the family therapist that the anger was an outcome of the frustration and despair of the family, which was being directed at society. Since "society" was an abstract form, the anger was focused on something concrete, such as the social workers from the Department of Social Services. When the supervisor helped the family therapist to define the source of the anger and to differentiate herself as a person from her role as the target of the anger, the family therapist's ability to accept the family returned and she could again focus on ways of helping them.

The supervisor can help family therapists and social workers become aware of the special role that they play in working with FED, that they are perceived as the representatives of "society" and therefore serve as the container for this population's anger. The ability of family therapists and social workers to accept this role, while distancing themselves, frees them for meeting the families' needs and for helping the families to work through their anger toward society. Parallel processes often occur between therapy and supervision. When such situations exist, the supervisor becomes the target of therapists' anger and frustration. Containing therapists' anger and frustration is often the first step in enabling therapists to work things through and once again be attuned to clients' needs.

COPING WITH A FAMILY'S OVERWHELMED CONDITION

The chaos of FED, characterized by the enormous amount of interconnected problems, creates an overwhelming situation for the therapeutic team in almost every therapeutic session. In many situations, family members cannot focus on the topic under discussion and constantly digress into complaining about other difficulties, usually expressing anger and blame as well. The number of problems and their intensity become an emotionally overwhelming condition for the family therapist and/or the therapeutic team. This is expressed by the feeling that "these kinds of difficulties should be solved immediately," as if it is an "all or nothing" situation. Such feelings are likely to lead to a sense of failure, frustration, anger, and, ultimately, burnout (Friesen and Sarros, 1981).

The goal of supervision in these situations is to help the family therapist and social worker to be empathic about the overwhelming context of the family, yet able to separate from it instead of being swallowed by it. Thus, it is sometimes the family therapist and/or the therapeutic team that has to do the rational analysis and present it to the family. The first stage in reaching this goal is to help the family therapist and/or the therapeutic team in separating themselves from the overwhelming situation. This can be achieved by asking the team to take a "time-out" in the therapeutic session in cases of life supervision, thus creating an immediate boundary within the therapeutic system between the team and the family. Sometimes, this "time-out" and the boundaries created provide sufficient space for team members to reorganize their feelings and directions. When this happens, the role of the supervisor is to offer the necessary support, which allows the team to reorganize. In some situations, it is also effective to suggest to team members that they share with the family their sense of being overwhelmed, and the difficulty of taking action in such a context, and invite family members to discuss how this overwhelming condition affects their daily lives.

If the family therapist, or the entire therapeutic team, cannot reorganize the overwhelming feelings and thoughts during the first stage, then the supervisor should move on to the second stage, during which concrete help is given to the supervisees. At this stage, the supervisee is asked to make a list of all the problems raised by the family, to define the intensity of each problem, and to assess which problems are urgent and which can be dealt with later, which problems can be used to get the family started, and which problems have a higher possibility of resolution and involve a shorter course of therapy. This type of analysis can be a guide for the therapist, who may choose to discuss it with the family as part of the therapeutic process. If the therapist determines that it would be too difficult for the family to undertake such an analysis, then the family therapist, or the case manager, can initiate it and suggest a direction to the family. This is demonstrated by the case of the Z. family:

> The family therapist came to a supervisory meeting after the therapeutic session, during which she and the entire therapeu-

tic team were overwhelmed by the enormous amount of problems and their intensity. In the supervisory session, time was first set aside to listen to the therapist's narration of the session. Based on the narrative, the supervisor summarized the problems that were mentioned by the family therapist and made a list. The list was given to the family therapist, who looked at it and immediately began to assess and evaluate the urgency and severity of the problems on the list, as well as the possibility of challenging the Z. family to cope with each one. The therapist indicated that this mode of summarizing the problems helped her to reorganize her thoughts and reduce her level of frustration. Furthermore, she projected that "if this list helped me, it might help the family too." Based on the supervision process, the family therapist returned to the family and shared her thoughts with them: "I and the entire team were stunned and shocked when we heard about all the problems you have been faced with. You, Mr. Z., are working very hard, but with your salary, you cannot provide for the needs of your family and are therefore frustrated. Mrs. Z. is depressed and helpless in taking care of her daily household chores because of lack of money and the difficulties in raising the children. Some of your children have been in various accidents; L., one of your daughters, is awaiting open-heart surgery, and B. and G. have dropped out of school. These are truly difficult problems. We, the team, have consulted with a colleague who was also shocked by the magnitude of the problems you are facing. We have been thinking that it is most important to help B. and G. return to school. It is important for the children themselves, but it also might help you and Mrs. Z. to know that the children are in school during the day. We would like to hear what you think about this suggestion." The therapist was not sure that the family was ready to analyze the situation to reach a concrete conclusion about the best course of action Thus, she conducted the analysis herself, but shared the process with the family and invited them to discuss the suggestion.

One may wonder whether by using this approach to cope with overwhelming conditions, we are not imposing the supervisor's view on the supervisees and then, in turn, encouraging them to impose it on FED. This might be the case when the supervisor perceives his or her understanding as the only correct one, but if this approach is seen merely as a basis for stimulating the reorganization of thoughts and feelings, then it is not a case of imposing one's authority on someone else. Furthermore, although many clients ask for concrete advice, they typically do not follow it. Rather, the advice given by the therapists, or, as the case may be, by the supervisors, serves to stimulate the problem-solving processes of the clients and the supervisees, leading to reorganization of their thoughts and feelings.

DEVELOPING A SYSTEMATIC VIEW RATHER THAN AN INDIVIDUAL PERSPECTIVE FOCUSED ON THE WIFE/MOTHER

In many of the relationships between female therapists and FED, we can observe a special identification of the wife with the therapist and/or social worker. Because a majority of husbands in FED are alcoholics and/or delinquents, and are violent toward their wives and children, the wives are perceived as victims. Most of the women in the FED population are responsible for rearing the children, doing the housework, and sometimes even working outside the home in order to contribute to the family's income. They have a certain amount of power within the family, which is based on their central role. This power is often enhanced by the attitude of others toward them as "the good" and their husbands as "the bad." In analyzing women's situation from a sociological, political, and legal perspective, it is obvious that changing laws and social norms can be effective in protecting women from abusive men and improving their social status. However, the perception of "good" and "bad" is damaging when trying to create changes within the family structure and its functioning. To help the family in the process of generating change, the husband should be allowed to join the family, even when he sometimes feels like an outsider and reverts to using pseudopower, that is, violence, to achieve his rightful place in the family.

In the supervisory process, it is essential to assist family therapists and social workers in minimizing their judgmental attitudes toward the husbands so that they do not maintain, or even worsen, the painful situation existing between the spouses. The majority of social workers and family therapists are women and, thus, more sensitive to gender issues concerning other women. This may possibly lead to extremely judgmental responses toward abusive, "irresponsible," and "dysfunctional" husbands, as well as toward the wife who ". . . continues to live with such a husband, instead of divorcing him." It is important to indicate that although there are many threats of divorce among FED, usually by the wives, these are generally not carried out; the women instead remain with their husbands (Sharlin, Shamai, and Gilad-Smolinsky, 1995). In the supervisory process, these ideological issues should be discussed in such a way that they are useful in creating change within the family, while allowing the therapists to remain loyal to their own set of beliefs. Let us illustrate this with the case of the A. family, as presented by the family's therapist:

> The family therapist reported that between the second and third meetings, Mr. A. had been violent at home. He yelled and broke furniture, and Mrs. A. called the police. Mr. A. was described as a handsome man who was unemployed, an alcoholic, and a drug addict also involved in drug pushing. Mrs. A. was described as a depressed woman who does not take care of herself, but tries very hard to function at home. During the first two meetings, the therapeutic team supported the wife against her husband's criticism. During supervision, the family therapist indicated that Mrs. A. always criticized her husband in front of the children, thus undermining his attempts to change. The supervisor assumed that the feeling of rejection had pushed Mr. A. to take his place in the family by force. Therefore, the family therapist was asked whether she had observed in Mr. A. any positive characteristics or behaviors. She said she had been able to identify Mr. A.'s commitment toward his children, as illustrated by his helping them with their homework. She also identified his cooking skills. The supervisor asked the therapist whether she could differentiate

between Mr. A. "the committed parent" and Mr. A. "the alcoholic and aggressor," and whether she could join with "the committed parent" side of Mr. A. despite his alcoholic and aggressive side. This was followed by a discussion on the therapist's feelings about criticizing a woman as opposed to criticizing a man and on the issue of violence and power being used in the family. As a result of this supervisory process, the family therapist joined Mr. A. and helped him to rejoin the family without aggression and criticism. This reduced his violent behavior, but it still took a long time for each of the spouses to give up the notion of Mr. A. as "the bad guy."

The supervisor must be aware of the tendency to follow a linear perspective, whereby each spouse is observed as an individual in a vacuum rather than through a systemic perspective. A supervisor should also understand that attitudes and behaviors have a contextual meaning and that they affect, and are affected by, each of the participants in the system.

RELATING TO THE ENTIRE TEAM

In the project described in this book, weekly supervision was given to the family therapist who was also the leader of the therapeutic team. Besides helping family therapists in their work with the families, supervision dealt with issues relating to processes within the team. Based on this experience, we strongly support weekly team supervision, especially if the case managers are also trained as family therapists, thereby challenging the role of the team leader. Team supervision reduces power and hierarchy issues, allowing open dialogue within a protective context, and enables working on parallel processes between the family and the team. However, it should be noted that processes within the team should be addressed for the benefit of the family in therapy and not for team-related purposes, which should be dealt with in a different setting.

TECHNIQUES IN SUPERVISION

During analysis of the supervisory sessions, we observed five main techniques that were most frequently used with FED. These techniques are often used in family therapy supervision, but they have a special meaning in the context of working with FED. These techniques are (1) ventilation, (2) reassurance, (3) focusing and setting boundaries, (4) guiding and directing, and (5) working on parallel processes between the therapeutic system and the therapist's own family system, as well as between the therapeutic system and the supervisory system.

Ventilation

The intensive work with FED exposes family therapists to painful experiences. These are related to the direct intervention with the family and to the leadership of the therapeutic team. Ventilation, which is very frequently used in both therapy and supervision, needs to be unconventional in supervising family therapists who work with FED. This means that the supervisor must be ready to listen to the family therapist beyond the supervisory sessions in cases that the therapist regards as urgent and overwhelming. As described in our project, one of the therapists used to contact the supervisor at the end of every day when she was working with the FED population. As the project progressed, her need to share with the supervisor beyond the supervisory sessions decreased and eventually disappeared. Another family therapist, who did not take advantage of the opportunity to share with the supervisor, was overwhelmed and decided to drop out of the project. The family therapist who replaced her was advised about the therapist's need for ventilation when working with FED and was encouraged to do so. She used this opportunity several times and found, too, that as she proceeded with the therapeutic process, her need to contact the supervisor beyond the supervisory sessions gradually declined.

The need for ventilation can be fulfilled by creating a supportive atmosphere among team members or in the agency. However, when the particular FED case is known as a very difficult one for the team and the other workers of the agency, ventilation can turn into a "coalition of despair," as described in Chapter 3. In such situations, it is useful to have a supervisor who does not know the family and who cannot join in aggressive, cynical jokes about the family or in the prevailing mood of hopelessness.

Reassurance

Because of the FED population's endless needs, many therapeutic techniques are required to deal with the problems. As a result, family therapists and social workers use various creative approaches, which are sometimes misunderstood or perceived as unprofessional by the management of some social services departments. Nevertheless, family therapists must have the courage to implement their plans and must get the reassurance they need to use creative methods in effecting change. Reassurance can be given by (1) integrating the specific direction chosen by the family therapist as part of the entire intervention, (2) helping the family therapist understand why it is sometimes difficult for the social agency and/or the family to join his or her direction, and (3) finding a way to rejoin with the social agency and/or the family by rebuilding and redeveloping the creative direction.

Focusing and Setting Boundaries

These techniques are used in helping family therapists remain flexible, while still being specific in defining the goal, the contract, and the therapeutic setting, as well as in implementing the therapeutic process according to its goal. It is very important to help therapists remain focused, to avoid drifting along with the family's impulsive behavior. When the therapist fails to focus and set clear-cut boundaries, the therapeutic process can easily degenerate into chaos, resulting in frustration that is shared by the family and the therapist alike.

Guiding and Directing

When a therapist expresses feelings of helplessness due to lack of skills, adequate intervention techniques, and therapeutic direction, the supervisor must offer assistance to the supervisee. The assistance is presented as creative thinking rather than as a "command" that the supervisee should obey and implement. This technique of supervision is effective when the supervisor's suggestion is examined according to the supervisee's own individual style of intervention and within the context of the specific family for whom guidance is needed. This technique is simmilar to "brainstorming," in that the supervisor and supervisee are working together to find suitable intervention directions in order to enrich the mode of reaching FED.

Working on Parallel Processes

Parallel processes exist between the therapeutic system (i.e., the therapist and the family) and the therapist's own family system, as well as between the therapeutic system and the supervisory system (i.e., the supervisor and supervisee). This process has to be clarified whenever the family therapist is "stuck" and cannot use the skills or direction given by the supervisor in working with the family. In such situations, it is possible that the therapeutic system and process evoke a resonance that belongs to the realm of the therapist's own family system, creating fear, anxiety, anger, or paralysis. When working on a parallel process, a systematic approach is utilized, with the understanding that both the family and the therapist affect and are affected by each other's feelings, emotions, memories, thoughts, and behaviors. It is important to understand what resonance the family evokes within the therapist and in what way. However, this resonance is only addressed within the context of therapy and not for the sake of the therapist.

Parallel processes can also occur between the therapeutic system and the supervisory system. The feelings of being overwhelmed, disorganized, frustrated, and angry can occur with supervisors as well, and in such cases, it is necessary to evaluate the effect of these feelings on the supervisory process. In most cases, supervisors will discover that through interaction with the supervisees, the therapeutic system can be better understood by creating a similar context. It is important to indicate this to the supervisees and to stress that after empathizing with the difficulty, one should separate from it. This should help supervisees to distance themselves in situations where they are drawn in by the family in distress.

In conclusion, supervision of family therapists and social workers who work with FED has the same goals as supervision of those working with other client populations. The additional goals relate to the overwhelming situations that often last for extended periods of time, causing the therapists' feelings of frustration and hopelessness. Such situations call for special ability on the part of the supervisor to contain these feelings and to turn them into hope. In this role, the supervisor is able to help therapists, who have become the target of FED's pain and anger, to distance themselves and to retain their freedom. This process requires the supervisor's attention to specific topics, as well as the creative use of conventional supervisory techniques.

PART V: THE RESEARCH PROJECT— PROCESS AND EVALUATION

Chapter 10

Developing a Project for Working with Families in Extreme Distress

The Ministry of Labor and Social Affairs in Israel approached the Center for Research and Study of the Family with a specific request: "to visit families in the Northern Region and attempt to identify strategies which could ameliorate their position." These families have historically been known to the Department of Social Services as "multiproblem," "hard to reach," "underorganized," and so on. In several instances, the apparently insurmountable nature of the family problems encountered had led social workers to give up hope of ending the cycle of despair. It seemed that every effort to deal with these families, to provide them with support, or to intervene on their behalf had been "torpedoed" by the families themselves. Above all, none of the workers' goals could be reached under the conditions that they found. Initial visits revealed poverty, illness, lack of adequate nutrition, and large outstanding debts, as well as neglect and abuse, total disorganization, lack of boundaries between family members, and despair. It appeared that every single facet of their lives was dysfunctional in one way or another. Indeed, health, personal hygiene, intellectual functioning, social and economic position, employment status, and standing in the community were all damaged or impaired.

First impressions of these families were difficult to bear and emotionally disheartening. It was clear that social workers often had difficulty in their attempts to ameliorate the position of such families, as each effort they invested seemed to be in vain. Thus, it was no surprise when a new mandate was issued, directing much closer observation of these families within the home setting to ascertain effective strategies for dealing with them. This approach allowed workers to establish the kind of in-depth relationships needed to accomplish positive results.

In one of our initial home visits, we met the R. family, which included Mr. and Mrs. R. and their two children, ages four and five. Mr. R., a thirty-year-old unemployed alcoholic, wanders aimlessly around the neighborhood. In the evening, he drinks heavily at the local pub. At midnight, he stumbles home, completely inebriated. Once home, his wife beats him and throws him out of the house, locking the iron entrance door. Wearing almost no clothing, Mr. R. is forced to spend the night on the ground at the entrance of his home. The two children witness how their mother treats their father and imitate her. When they walk by him, they, too, strike him and push him out of the way. The four-year-old takes a rubber knife, approaches Mr. R., and moves his hand back and forth, pretending to stab his father. The R. home reeks with the smell of urine and feces. The bathroom has no door because it has long been broken and since removed. At 10 a.m., the five-year-old emerged, eating her breakfast: a dried-up piece of bread. The mother commented that she had no food to feed the children. She added that she was unable to clean the house because as soon as she finished cleaning one room, the children messed it up again.

Our profile revealed that Mr. R. had previously been employed in a local factory, had been satisfied with his job, and had been earning enough money to maintain a regular family life. As the result of an unfortunate work accident in which a heavy cart fell on him, he became disabled, lost his job, and shortly thereafter began to drink. Although he does receive disability benefits, Mr. R. spends the majority of the money on alcohol. Only a paltry sum remains for his wife and family. After discovering Mr. R.'s interest in animals during the course of our interview, we recommended that the social worker assigned to the case find a position for Mr. R. at the local zoo. Upon making such an arrangement, the worker found that the new position had an immediate effect on Mr. R. The additional income, combined with the sense of self-worth fostered by employment in a field of his choice, brought about a fundamental change in Mr. R.'s life. He was able to request the help he needed in restoring his relationship with his wife and children. The couple was then invited to join therapy, an offer that was gladly accepted by Mr. R.

Mrs. R. was initially hesitant, but then agreed, as a result of the trust that had already been established.

From our home visits, we concluded that gaining access to the clients' home as a team enabled us to view the situation from a variety of perspectives. This allowed us to examine the dynamics of the family as a whole and consequently provided us with the vital information needed to devise solutions for their multiple problems.

THE PILOT FED PROJECT

The Department of Social Services represented the field agency, hosted the project, and supplied the families. Each family was visited at home by a team, consisting of the directors of both centers, who served as family therapists with different backgrounds in training, orientation, and experience; a social worker from the Department of Social Services, who was assigned to the case; and the regional supervisor of the Ministry of Labor and Social Affairs.

The families we visited were first approached by the social workers from the Department of Social Services. Prior to our home visits, these workers were involved in what we called "previsits," which effectively prepare the families for subsequent meetings. They provided the families with an overview of the project and its purpose, as well as an explanation of the role of "the University people" in helping the Department of Social Services to address the families' needs. Each family was asked to sign a confidential release form and to provide consent to videotape the session for research purposes. We encountered no refusals or hesitation on the part of the clients, who were generally very cooperative and ready to "help us help others in the future." Before visiting each family, the team met for a briefing led by the social worker who provided basic information on the family's sociodemographic structure, its history with the Department of Social Services, and details on how the family was treated prior to the commencement of the project.

Since most families came from the traditional patriarchal background, we found it useful to respect that culture and, hence, allowed the father to be the first respondent. Once inside the home, we asked the head of the family to introduce other members and to elucidate some of the family's most pressing problems. We then turned to the spouses, asking them to complete the picture and to share their views on the family. Finally, we asked each of the children to do the same. Much to our surprise, the families were very willing to participate and able to contribute valuable information to the family story.

By the end of the pilot study, we were operating under the assumption that each family has a separate and unrelated history, bearing little resemblance to the dynamics of other families. However, as we delved further into the project, it became increasingly clear to us that family units did, in fact, share many common patterns, in spite of any idiosyncratic differences among them.

Most of the couples who took part in the pilot study were between the ages of thirty-five and forty-five. The majority of families were second-generation North African immigrants, characteristically possessing inadequate education and often not even having completed elementary school. None of the parents had a profession or even any specific training, and many were unemployed. The bulk of their income came either from disability or family benefits. They married young and had an average of six to eight children. Their children had multiple problems, including poor functioning at school, emotional problems, and attempts at suicide.

Most of the men had a chronic disease, were drug users or alcoholics, beat their spouses, and/or had a history of criminal behavior, often having spent time in prison. They generally appeared hopeless and displayed low self-esteem and poor verbal functioning. In terms of physical appearance, they looked generally unkempt, and it was not uncommon for them to have rotten teeth and to show other signs of neglected personal hygiene.

The women in these families projected a stronger image and possessed a higher level of verbal functioning than their husbands. They often appeared as dominant, carrying the burden of maintaining the household on their shoulders, in addition to caring for the children and dealing with other family problems. However, for many of them, this image appeared to be a facade. In fact, the women usually had a history of running away from home, displaying rebellious and impulsive behavior, and being heavy drinkers. Nevertheless, most of them appeared to be young and well groomed. Perhaps the large number of children and household responsibilities contributed to the mistaken conclusion that these women were more in control than their husbands.

As we completed our observations at the conclusion of the pilot study, we gave each of the workers both our short- and long-term recommendations. Included was advice on how to proceed with the family as a unit and as individual members. The pilot study generated the following findings and recommendations:

1a. *Finding:* Social workers involved with FED may have very little current and valid knowledge about the family. The gap between what is known to the worker and the real state of the family results in a lack of vital information needed for appropriate assessment and treatment.

1b. *Recommendation:* Workers must focus on goal-oriented data collection, based on valid documents or legal certificates. In gathering data, workers must be active in raising questions as well as in clarifying related details. Most families do not object to providing information if the matter is clearly explained.

2a. *Finding:* These families manifest high levels of disorganization, lack of clear boundaries, and role confusion. The couple system and/or the parental system is significantly impaired and suffers from difficulties in communication. Husbands appear weak in comparison to the pseudostoicism of the women.

2b. *Recommendation:* Workers must facilitate the process of establishing clear boundaries, clarifying roles, and strengthening the husbands' abilities to take a more active role in family affairs rather than resorting to violence.

3a. *Finding:* Couples engage in almost no family planning and take little responsibility in raising their children.

3b. *Recommendation:* It is important to challenge these families to participate in a family planning program and to learn to assume a more mature outlook in terms of the responsibilities of raising children.

4a. *Finding:* These families live below the poverty line and depend on governmental support. Most have heavy debts and lack basic knowledge of how to balance a budget.
4b. *Recommendation:* It is useful to instruct families in budgeting strategies.

5a. *Finding:* As families in a state of extreme distress, they suffer from major problems in basic functioning areas, such as social skills, economics, health, and so forth. As time goes on, their problems become more complex, making early intervention and prevention measures that much harder to implement.
5b. *Recommendation:* An immediate intervention must be initiated by several workers to combat multiple family problems and to avoid the internalization of despair on the part of the individual case worker. Several specific directions for intervention are recommended here: creating hope for change; developing an effort to generate resources (both internal and external) to be used for change; and clarifying and defining roles in the family structure.

Upon conclusion of the pilot project, our future aim was twofold: to continue the project with FED more systematically and to examine all of the aforementioned findings and recommendations.

THE FED PROJECT

The design and execution of the FED project was a direct and natural extension of the FED pilot study—namely, the development of a model and the guiding principles for helping the Department of Social Services' team deal with FED. In addition, it allowed for the formulation and testing of interventions suitable for coping with FED. All of this was to be achieved through additional skilled staff to be supported by a training and teaching system.

The project was designed to be carried out in two communities, in two different social services departments. The project goals were delineated as follows:

1. To undertake an innovative demonstration project with families regarded as FED
2. To integrate intervention systems and resources so as to induce a planned change
3. To develop a working model for intervention such as an FED Center at the Department of Social Services

To accomplish these goals, our plan followed three principles:

1. The therapeutic sessions would be conducted by a team to avoid worker burnout. The team should meet before and after each session to review, summarize, and plan the next meeting, as well as to provide one another with feedback. The team is to be composed of three workers with different roles, as follows (see Figure 10.1):
   - A social worker who is also an expert family therapist will serve as the team leader in charge of conducting the therapeutic meetings with the family and providing the family and team members with specific tasks.
   - A social worker from the Department of Social Services, who is the permanent worker assigned to the family, will serve as the case manager. The social worker's role is to provide the family with necessary aid, establish a support system, link the family with community institutions, coordinate the multiprofessional team, monitor the family during the "rest" period, and provide continuity of care once the project is completed.
   - A social work aide, usually a second-year MSW student, will serve as the project coordinator. The project coordinator arranges and coordinates the therapeutic meetings, acts as an observer during therapy sessions, assumes a cotherapist's role when needed, and provides feedback to the team. In addition, the project coordinator's responsibilities are as a researcher involved in data collection; administration of the relevant questionnaires to family members, both before and after intervention; and arrangements for audio- and videotaping the therapeutic meetings.
2. The process must be planned, focused, have clear goals, and cover a limited time period. Our plan included ten ninety-minute

therapeutic sessions. Each meeting was planned so that the clients and the workers could envision some change within a foreseeable time frame in order to strengthen their hope and produce immediate satisfaction. The limited time period, usually three months, was to be followed by a three-month period without meetings, providing the family with the space to reflect and to practice the homework that they had been assigned. The second phase to follow would consist of ten more therapeutic meetings, thereby creating an overall treatment-rest-treatment model.

3. The therapeutic sessions must be conducted at the family's home so as to reduce the possibility of manipulation and the workers' uncertainty regarding whether the family will attend. Otherwise, such uncertainty constitutes a major source of frustration in these cases and serves to exacerbate preexisting suspicion and distrust. Furthermore, meeting the family on home territory yields important therapeutic information in a process that is fostered by observing people in their natural environment.

FIGURE 10.1. The Therapeutic Team

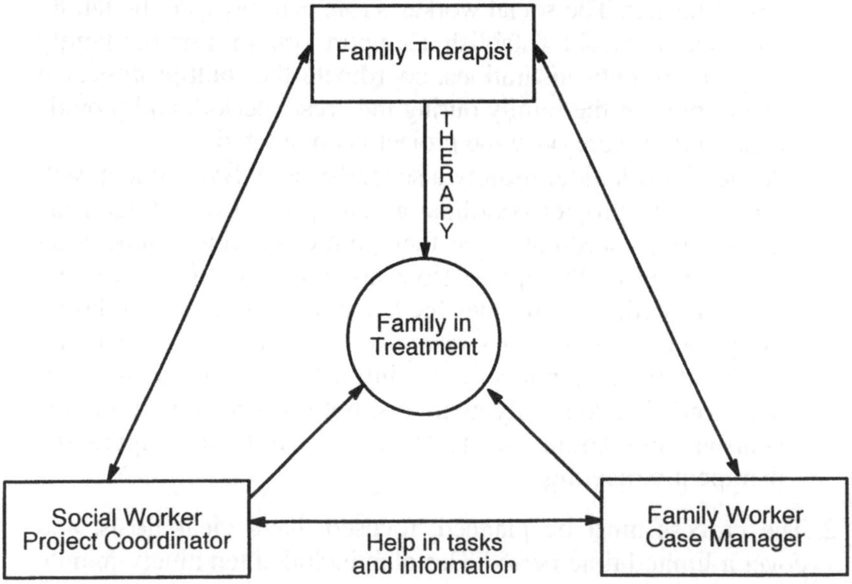

METHOD AND PROCEDURE

Each social services department provided twenty of the "most difficult families" on their rosters. Ten families were selected randomly from each of the two participating communities to be placed in the research group, while the remaining twenty families formed the control group. We found that the families who participated in the project had characteristics similar to those involved in the pilot study. The average FED family was composed of a forty-year-old husband and a thirty-four-year-old wife. Seventy-five percent of husbands and wives were of North African origin. Most of their lives had been spent in Israel, having emigrated between the ages of four and six. They were from traditional religious sects, and their educational level was seventh or eighth grade. Seventy-five percent of the couples were from second-generation FED families. Most of the couples had debts, and half of them were unemployed. Fifty percent were diagnosed with physical and/or mental health problems. The average time of cohabitation was fifteen years, and the mean number of children was six. Half of the couples cited either out-of-wedlock pregnancies or arranged marriages as reasons for their unions. All couples reported several periods of separation from each other.

In each social services department (one in each community), the social workers (case managers) were responsible for the recruitment of the twenty families and the random assignment of ten of them to the research group. The social workers invited each family to their Department of Social Services, where the goals of the project were explained. Social workers stated that they would like to share the families' difficulties with them to find out how they coped and struggled with their problems and to learn how these hardships could be reduced or overcome. The families were informed about the therapeutic meetings to be held at their homes and were asked to sign a written agreement acknowledging their decision to participate in the project. They were introduced to the project coordinator, who administered a battery of questionnaires. The twenty families composing the control group were told that their part in the project would only involve the completion of surveys, which might be helpful to the worker in future meetings (though they did receive regular agency services as needed). The twenty families in the research group were instructed that the case manager would make arrangements to meet them in their homes once a week for the duration of ten sessions. They were assured that all the sessions would be videotaped for research purposes only and were promised full confidentiality. Written consent was obtained in each case.

Special attention was given to professional growth and development. Six teaching and training days were planned and carried out during the project. On the first day, all teams were told about the goals of intervention, as well as the overall strategy. The entire project staff continued to meet every two weeks for a teaching and training day, providing the workers with a vehicle for reporting back to the group on their contacts with the families, presenting case conferences, and raising specific issues.

Treatment sessions were evaluated and planned. In cases requiring a multiprofessional team, one was organized by the case manager to join the FED intervention team for coordinating treatment efforts. This multiprofessional team consisted of community members with whom the family interacted, such as family physicians, nurses, teachers, school headmasters, and lawyers. The specific composition of each multiprofessional team varied according to the needs of the particular family and the outcome being sought. The team, directed by the project coordinator and supervised by the family therapist, was responsible for sharing information relevant to the family's problems, prioritizing needs, and advocating on behalf of the family with community agencies.

The Regional Center for Family Therapy Training and Intervention provided ongoing supervision to the family therapist at a minimum of once every two weeks and, if needed, more frequently.

As one might expect, there are always discrepancies between the planning of a project and its execution. While the strategy was quite clear to us, the day-to-day dynamics made every step unique and challenging. How does one begin to get such a big wheel rolling? Even after the accomplishment of setting a multiphase project in motion, which depends on the effective cooperation of so many diverse groups, unforeseeable obstacles remain. We now turn our attention to the logistics of the commencement of the project, as well as to some of these obstacles (see Figure 10.2).

FIGURE 10.2. Logistics of the Project

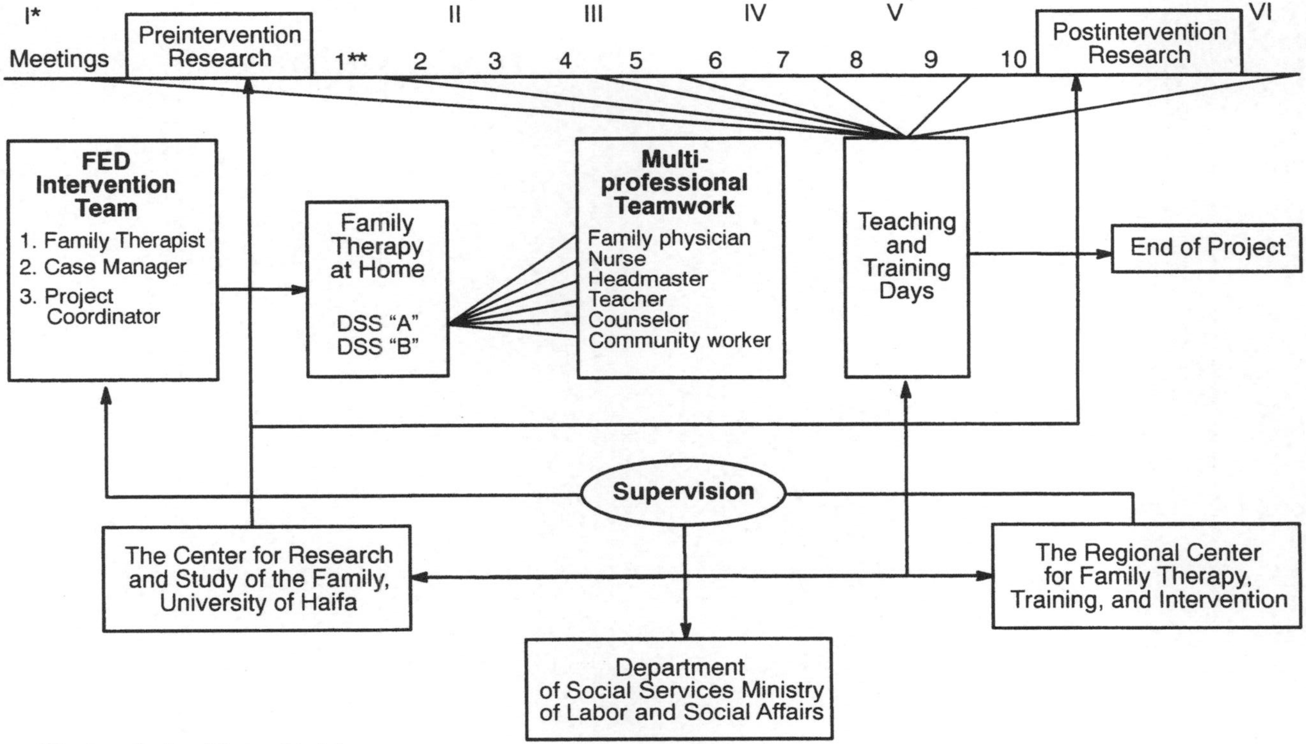

*Six days for teaching and training.
**Ten sessions of intervention with each family.

Chapter 11

Pre- and Postproject Measurements and Evaluation

Ever since therapy was aimed at reducing problems and psychic pain, scientists have attempted to measure its success and outcome. For those who believed that eliminating the symptoms meant a return to normality, then identifying the symptoms heralded success. Therapists simply reported on a successful intervention by virtue of the disappearance of the symptoms. Thus, symptom free meant "healthy" or "normal." For others, relieving the symptoms is not the core of therapy, as they focus on the actual experience of the individual and the family in therapy, which, in itself, creates a new perception about life. These two diverse viewpoints lead to different kinds of evaluation, as well as to different definitions of therapeutic effectiveness.

The scientific approach to social work practice, as well as family therapy, is very meaningful. Kurt Lewin once said that without a theory, we crawl, and with a theory, we run. Hence, by basing our progress on empirical data and scientific methods, we can attempt to contribute new concepts for practical intervention.

Reid (1987) suggests that using the scientific method may serve as a framework for social work practice, even though such practice is considered an art form. This kind of scientific orientation, Reid further notes, requires the use of terms and concepts, which are clearly connected to empirical events. Therefore, systematic data collection, careful drawing of conclusions, and consideration of alternative explanations will ensure more responsible utilization of our knowledge, based on research (Reid and Smith, 1981). Polansky (1986) points out six important functions that a good theory may serve in practice, the first of which is providing a frame of reference before acting. This gives workers a feeling of knowledge and serves as a systemic influence on their efforts, enabling them to focus attention on the data at hand and to transmit their treatment experience to others. Finally, it helps workers to maintain their self-discipline and professional approach, thereby enabling them to examine the efficiency of their interventions.

From the beginning of our project, we faced a major dilemma. On the one hand, we could not present a major study or an innovative project without attempting to measure its results. One cannot claim effectiveness in any intervention without the ability to show what progress has been made and what has changed. On the other hand, evaluating a clinical intervention raises both objective and subjective problems: How do we evaluate and measure change objectively? Which instrument could be used, and how? No less important, does the measurement in itself influence the project? When assessing FED, one should bear in mind the complexity of utilizing research methods with this population. The instrument and procedure used must be carefully chosen and executed, based on subjects that are relevant to the FED reality. A brief illustration will suffice: FED cannot be asked questions regarding "saving money" or "using credit cards." Such questions are often asked in studies of Western cultures and are suitable mainly for the middle class. The same can be said about the language used with FED. This chapter will describe our efforts to overcome these two issues by presenting our objective measurements in the quantitative part of the study and the findings that emerged, as well as the qualitative part and its findings.

THE STUDY POPULATION

The following criteria were used for selecting the families:

1. Families that include the father, the mother, and their children (from the parents' first or second marriage)
2. Families that had been known to the Department of Social Services for a long period of time
3. Multiproblem families, that is, those with no specific type or number of problems

4. Families that, up to the time of the study, had been unable to improve their functioning
5. Families that could not be helped by the social worker on the case (who gave up on them, stating, "I do not know what to do")

Although we planned to include forty families in our study, the final usable sample consisted of only thirty-five families, of which seventeen were undergoing treatment and eighteen were included in the control group. Both the study and the control group were taken from two separate departments at the Department of Social Services. The sample of thirty-five clients was randomly divided into study and research groups. No significant differences were found between the two groups at the first measurement before the project started.

Sociodemographic characteristics of the entire sample are presented in Table 11.1. The mean age of the men was forty-two. Two-thirds of the men were born in Morocco and had immigrated to Israel. With the majority having a total of seven years in school, 30 percent had no reading or writing ability and an additional 40 percent had difficulty with reading or writing. About half of the sample had lived and was educated outside the parental home before the age of eighteen. Nearly 60 percent of the men had served in the compulsory Israeli Defense Forces, either full- or part-time.

As for the women, their mean age was thirty-five. Second-generation Israeli women, born to fathers who had emigrated from Morocco, represented half of the sample. Half of the women had had up to eight years of schooling, but had difficulty with reading and writing. The majority of the women had lived with their parents until the age of eighteen, and none had served in the armed forces, although service is compulsory for women as well. Women's mean age at the time of marriage was 20.5 ($SD = 3.86$), while men's average age was 27.39 ($SD = 9.01$). In general, women married between the ages of fifteen and twenty, and men married between twenty-one and thirty.

The mean number of years of marriage at the time of the study was 14.21 ($SD = 6.67$), and 69 percent of the couples had married either because of pregnancy or parental pressure (see Table 11.2). This was the second marriage for only 3 percent of the women and 15 percent of the men. More than half of the couples had unstable

TABLE 11.1. Sample Distribution of Men and Women According to Sociodemographic Variables

		Men		Women	
Variable	**Value**	**%**	**N**	**%**	**N**
Country of subject's birth	Israel	27.3	9	54.5	18
	Morocco	63.6	21	42.4	14
	Other Mideast countries	9.1	3	3.0	1
Country of subject's father's birth	Morocco	75.7	25	63.6	21
	Other Mideast countries	24.3	8	36.4	12
Age	23-30 years old	6.1	2	24.2	8
	31-40	48.5	16	54.5	18
	41-50	33.3	11	21.2	7
	51 and up	12.1	4	—	—
Resided until age 18	Parental home	54.5	18	87.9	29
	Outside parental home	45.5	15	12.1	4
Military service	Never drafted	36.4	12	97.0	32
	Partial service	27.2	9	—	—
	Full service	36.4	12	3.0	1
Ability to read and write in Hebrew	Does not read or write	30.3	10	33.3	11
	With difficulty	39.4	13	39.4	13
	No difficulty	30.3	10	27.3	9
Additional training	No training	30.3	10	54.5	18
	Has had training	69.7	23	45.5	15

marital relations, which included periods of separation or even the beginning of divorce proceedings.

Table 11.2 clearly reveals the unstable nature of these marriages. Nearly three-quarters of the families have been in treatment offered by the Department of Social Services. The mean number of children is 4.76 (SD = 1.17), and 72 percent of the families have four children or more. The total number of children in our sample was 170, with 96 percent of them living together with their parents.

Characteristics of the distress level are presented in Table 11.3. Most of the women and 60 percent of the men do not work, and 83 percent are heavily indebted. One-half of our sample was found

TABLE 11.2. Sample Distribution of the Marital System in Percentages

Variable	Value	%	N
Number of years married	3-5	15.2	5
	6-10	18.2	6
	11-15	30.3	10
	15-26	36.4	12
Marital back-ground	Pregnancy	34.5	10
	Parental pressure	34.5	10
	Romantic love	31.0	9
Marital stability	No separation or divorce	45.5	15
	Separation period / filed for divorce	54.5	18
Number of years in DSS treatment	1-5	24.2	8
	6-10	33.3	11
	11-26	42.4	14
Religiousness	Orthodox	21.2	7
	Traditional	66.7	22
	Observers	12.1	4

TABLE 11.3. Sample Distribution According to Variables Characterized by a High Level of Distress

		Men		Women	
Variable	Value	%	N	%	N
Employment situation	No work	60.6	20	84.8	28
	When work is available	12.1	4	6.1	2
	Permanent work	27.3	9	9.1	3
Physical health	Healthy	48.5	16	42.4	14
	Not healthy	51.5	17	57.6	19
Mental health	No psychiatric hospitalization	87.9	29	87.9	29
	Some psychiatric hospitalization	12.1	4	12.1	4
Reporting on depression	Not depressed	45.5	15	39.4	13
	Depressed	54.5	18	60.6	20
Suicidal attempts	No attempts	81.8	27	78.8	26
	Several attempts	18.2	6	21.2	7
Rage and anger	None	27.3	9	21.2	7
	Some	72.7	24	78.8	26
Alcoholism	None	54.5	18	100.0	33
	Some	45.5	15	—	0
Drug abuse	None	72.7	24	97.0	32
	Some	27.3	9	3.0	1
Jail period	Never been to jail	78.8	26	97.0	32
	Has been to jail	21.2	7	3.0	1

to be in poor health and depressed. One-fifth had attempted suicide, and more than two-thirds of the men and the women experienced outbreaks of rage and anger. Half of the men were alcoholics, nearly one-third were addicted to drugs, and 21 percent had served various jail terms. Additional data revealed that in one-third of the families, one child had serious health problems and that in 12 percent of the families, more than two children had serious health problems. In 64 percent of the families, children had learning difficulties. The FED in our study represent multiproblem families with severe physical and mental health problems affecting their social and family functioning.

THE QUANTITATIVE ANALYSIS

In the literature, little attention has been given to the evaluation of treatment with FED using objective research instruments for empirical studies. Also, the criteria for successful intervention or some improvement of functioning are frequently omitted. Some studies report on improvement in family functioning based on a description of the intervention process with one family (Craig and Hurry, 1981; Hardy-Fanta and MacMahon-Herrera, 1981; Levine, 1964; Tomlinson and Peters, 1981). The reader will recall the review of the literature on intervention in Chapter 2. As mentioned, few studies can be cited to support the results of a given intervention. From our pilot study, we have learned that FED have two things in common: (1) impaired family functioning, as measured by the McMaster Family Assessment Device (FAD), and (2) impaired family structure, as measured by the Kvebaek Family Sculpture Technique (KFST).

Family Functioning

Family functioning was measured by the McMaster FAD. This instrument was developed by Epstein, Baldwin, and Bishop (1983); Epstein, Bishop, and Baldwin (1982); Miller and associates (1985); and Grotevant and Carlson (1989). The purpose of the instrument is to assess the various dimensions of family functioning to improve the work of researchers and practitioners in their study and treatment of the family. The instrument was designed to help differentiate between a healthy and an unhealthy family.

The Family Assessment Device includes seven dimensions of family functioning. The original six dimensions of family functioning covered are problem solving, communication, roles, affective responsiveness, affective involvement, and behavior control. A seventh dimension was subsequently added: general functioning. The version of the Family Assessment Device used in the present study included fifty-three items. Subjects were asked to choose among four answers from "absolutely agree" to "absolutely disagree." The score was calculated for each spouse individually, ranging from 1.00, healthy functioning, to 4.00, unhealthy functioning. The lower the score, the better the family functioning. Internal consistency, as reported by the authors of the instrument, ranged between .72 and .92, and test-retest reliability between .66 and .76 (Miller et al., 1985; Grotevant and Carlson, 1989). Other validity tests, such as "concurrent validity," and correlation with "Family Unit Inventory," "Faces II," and "Social Desirability," have yielded positive results, showing that the instrument is useful for researchers and clinicians in providing information on family functioning dimensions, without being influenced by social desirability.

In Table 11.4 and Figure 11.1, we can observe the means and standard deviations of the men and women at the time of the first measurement before the intervention began.

Examination of Table 11.5 reveals that the means of all the dimensions are relatively high; namely, impaired family functioning is evident among all the families in our study. To test whether there were differences between the men and the women in our sample in the various dimensions, we performed the paired t-test (see Table 11.4). No significant differences were found between the genders in the seven dimensions of the Family Assessment Device.

To determine whether there were significant differences between the experimental and the control groups before the beginning of the intervention, we performed a one-way MANOVA. No significant differences were found between the experimental and the control groups. Our major hypothesis was that the effect of our inter-

TABLE 11.4. Means and Standard Deviations of Husbands and Wives in the Dimensions of Family Functioning, As Measured Before the Intervention

	Women N = 30		Men N = 30		
Dimension	**Mean**	**SD**	**Mean**	**SD**	**T = Value**
Problem solving	2.38	0.55	2.35	0.60	0.27
Communication	2.52	0.48	2.65	0.62	1.11
Roles	2.64	0.68	2.41	0.64	1.46
Affective responsiveness	2.44	0.62	2.50	0.66	0.35
Affective involvement	2.91	0.49	2.95	0.50	0.30
Control	2.29	0.49	2.39	0.45	0.91
General functioning	2.00	0.64	2.35	0.81	1.88

FIGURE 11.1. Comparison Between Husbands and Wives in the Dimension of Family Functioning Before the Intervention (Mean Score)

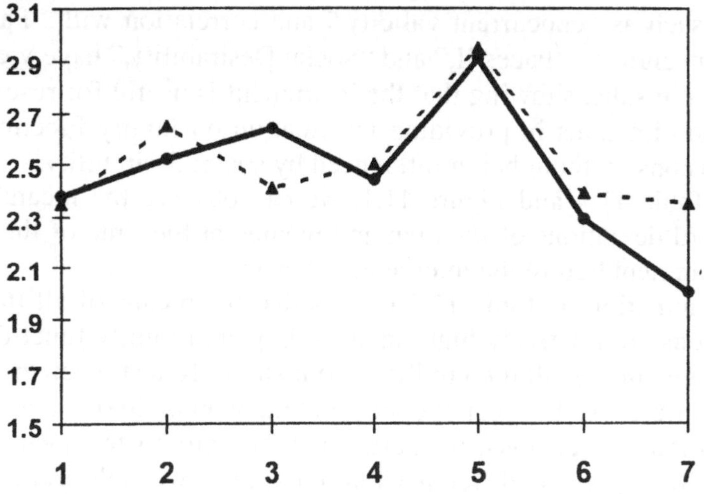

1. Problem Solving
2. Communication
3. Roles
4. Affective Responsiveness
5. Affective Involvement
6. Control
7. General Functioning

TABLE 11.5. Means and Standard Deviations of the Men and Women of Both Treatment and Control Groups in the Family Functioning Dimensions, Before and After the Intervention

			Problem Solving		Commu-nication		Roles		Affective Respon-siveness		Affective Involve-ment		Control		General Function-ing	
	Gender	Time Measured	$\bar{X}$	SD	$\bar{X}$	SD	$\bar{X}$	SD	$\bar{X}$	SD	$\bar{X}$	SD	$\bar{X}$	SD	$\bar{X}$	SD
EXPERIMENT Gp. N = 11	Women	Before	2.43	.43	2.39	.44	2.38	..58	2.27	.59	2.92	.49	2.22	.39	1.91	.72
	Women	After	2.30	.38	2.24	.45	2.42	.72	2.56	.64	2.59	.46	2.13	.32	2.40	.52
	Men	Before	2.55	.41	2.52	.58	2.49	.63	2.48	.37	3.05	.54	2.44	.47	2.66	.62
	Men	After	2.33	.42	2.54	.45	2.34	.56	2.40	.54	2.59	.38	2.40	.35	2.40	.55
CONTROL Gp. N = 14	Women	Before	2.52	.55	2.58	.57	2.86	.69	2.48	.72	2.96	.54	2.45	.53	2.31	.48
	Women	After	2.67	.49	2.72	.58	2.94	.71	2.53	.53	3.17	.47	2.35	.48	2.46	.52
	Men	Before	2.27	.75	2.78	.60	2.40	.69	2.40	.81	2.87	.51	2.34	.41	2.32	.96
	Men	After	2.44	.78	2.74	.47	2.34	.95	2.70	.47	2.65	.63	2.22	.36	2.43	.85
Interaction Treatment × Time			5.50	.49	.10	.07	6.31	.06	.00							
Interaction Treatment × Time × Sex			.25		1.33		.01		3.47		.98		.07		3.88	

vention program with FED would become apparent by the experimental group families' noticeable improvement in their family functioning at the end of the treatment.

Table 11.5 presents the means and standard deviations of the experiment and control groups as measured "before" and "after" intervention. No improvement was found in the control group between the two measurements. Variance analysis yielded significant improvement within the treatment group, both in the problem solving and affective involvement dimensions, as compared with the control group ("problem solving" $=(F[1,21])=5.50$, $p<.05$; "affective involvement" $=(F[1,21]=6.31$, $p.<05)$. The results can be seen in Figures 11.2 and 11.3. Figure 11.2 relates to the problem-solving dimension, demonstrating an unexplainable drop in the ability to solve problems in the control group, while there was an improvement in problem-solving skills in the experimental group following treatment.

Figure 11.3 shows a similar direction in the affective involvement dimension, namely, an improvement in the experimental group and no change in the control group. Thus, we can assume that the intervention with FED was effective in enhancing problem-solving skills and affective involvement.

When examining the age of the subjects in relation to family functioning, we found a negative correlation for both men and women. Thus, as the subject ages, his or her family functioning worsens. Among women, this decrease in functioning appears in the problem-solving dimension, and among men, in the dimensions of general functioning and affective involvement. Both men and women showed a negative correlation between the number of children and family functioning. The more children a woman had, the poorer her problem-solving skills, whereas the men scored poorly in the roles dimension.

Family Structure

Family structure was measured by the Kvebaek Family Sculpture Technique (KFST), developed by David Kvebaek in Norway in 1973. The instrument was developed in response to the difficulty clinicians experience in remembering the various structures and interactions in groups of families (Cromwell, Fournier, and Kvebaek,

FIGURE 11.2. Mean Scores of Problem-Solving Dimension in Family Functioning Among Treatment Group and Control Group, Before and After Intervention

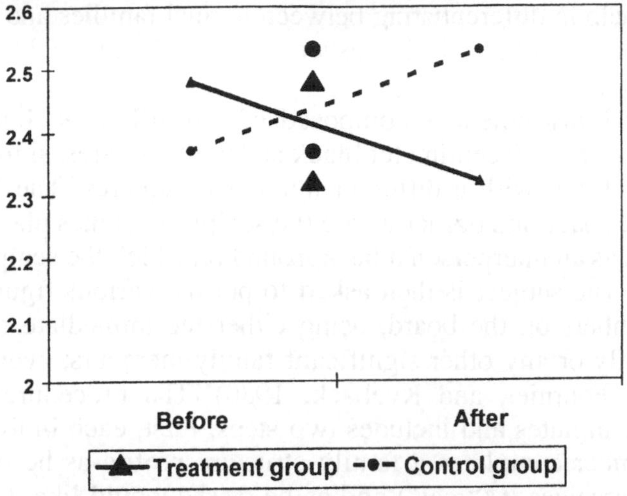

FIGURE 11.3. Mean Scores of Affective Involvement Dimensions in Family Functioning Among Treatment Group and Control Group, Before and After Intervention

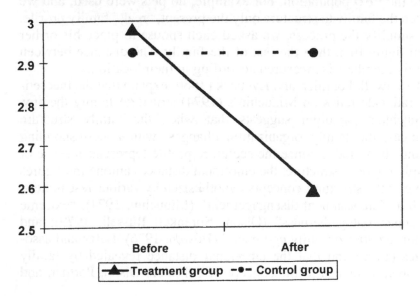

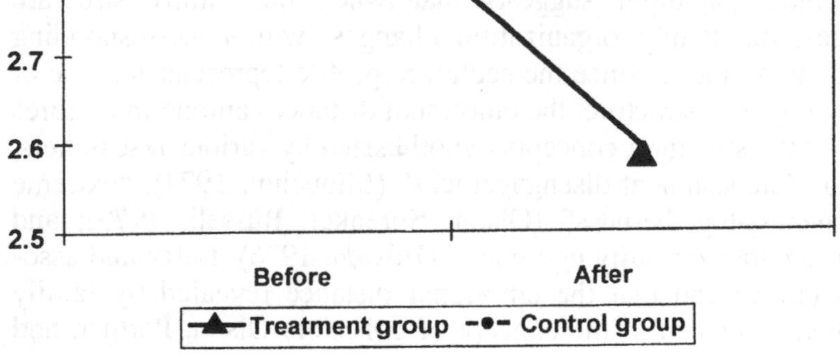

1980). The KFST has been used by many clinicians, as well as in empirical studies demonstrating that people are able to give a spatial presentation to important interpersonal relationships. Such a presentation can help in differentiating between normal families and those with various types of physical or psychosocial problems (Ecklad and Vandvik, 1992).

The KFST instrument is composed of a board, 1 × 1 meter, divided into 10 × 10 centimeter black and white squares, similar to a chessboard, but with a different number of squares. The board signifies the space and border where the sculpturing takes place and is thus used as an interpersonal background on which the sculptures are placed. The subject is then asked to put the various figures of family members on the board, using either the immediate or extended family or any other significant family members, even pets (Cromwell, Fournier, and Kvebaek, 1980). The procedure lasts about thirty minutes and includes two steps. First, each individual family member completes a family structure profile as he or she presently perceives it ("real") and as he or she would like it to be ("ideal"). Second, all family members are asked to reach a consensus of both the real and ideal family profile. In our research, we moderated the procedure and adopted a few changes to accommodate the FED population. For example, no pets were used, and we asked the family to structure only the present, "real," family profile. To simplify the process, we asked each spouse to place his or her own figure first, then the rest of the family. The distance between family members is measured according to their location.

Cromwell, Fournier, and Kvebaek (1980) explain that the theoretical rationale relies on Minuchin's (1974) structural family therapy. Minuchin's paradigm suggests that when the family structure changes, the family organization changes, with a corresponding change in attitudes. Since the sculpture profile represents a sense of family relations structure, the emotional distances among the figures serve as the structural concepts hypothesized by various researchers, such as "enmeshment-disengagement" (Minuchin, 1974); "extreme separateness-togetherness" (Olson, Sprenkel, Russell, 1979); and "undifferentiated family ego mass" (Bowen, 1976). Berry and associates (1990) add that the emotional distance revealed by family members is related to the concept of cohesion. Olson, Portner, and

Lavee (1985) defined cohesion as the emotional connection between family members, or the degree to which family members are connected to their family.

For the analysis of the data revealed by the KFST, we followed the procedure suggested by Ecklad and Vandvik (1992): the higher the score, the greater the distance. Since we hypothesized that there would be a change in family structure, as measured before and after the intervention, we calculated a different score for each subject. Positive scores show an increase in the distance (divergence), or an increase in scatteredness. Negative scores show a drop in the distance (convergence), or a drop in scatteredness. When the distance changes, it is important to find out whether, clinically, it is in the desired direction, that is, whether enmeshed families will increase the distance and scatteredness, while disengaged families will decrease it.

In our project, we asked both the husband and wife to place their family members on the board. To test the changes in family structure, as measured before and after the intervention, we measured the distances between the spouses, between the couple and the children, and between the couple and other significant members of the extended family. Altogether, there were ten dimensions, measured as follows: (1 and 2) distance from the mother/father to the farthest child; (3 and 4) distance from the mother/father to the closest child; (5 and 6) distance from the mother/father to the children; (7 and 8) scatteredness of mother/father and children; (9) distance between spouses; (10) distance of spouses from extended family.

Differences in the measurement of distances, before and after the intervention, were calculated. Mann-Whitney nonparametrical analysis was used to test for differences between the experimental and control groups, before and after the intervention. No significant differences were found between the groups before the intervention. However, after the intervention, significant differences were found between the two groups in two KFST dimensions: the distance between the couple and the extended family and the distance between the mother and children (see Table 11.6).

The data reveal that in the treatment group, the distances between the mother and the children and between the couple and the extended family were found to be smaller than in the control group, as

TABLE 11.6. Dimensions of Family Structure (KFST) Mean of Differences Between Treatment and Control Groups

	Treatment Group N = 11	Control Group N = 14	U
Distance between couple and extended family	8.91	16.21	32.0***
Distance between the spouses	14.50	11.82	60.5
Scatteredness of father and children	12.18	13.64	68.0
Distance of father from children	11.55	14.14	61.0
Distance between father and closest child	11.91	12.08	65.0
Distance between father and farthest child	12.65	10.54	48.5
Scatteredness between mother and children	10.45	15.00	49.0
Distance of mother from children	9.82	15.50	42.0*
Distance of mother from closest child	14.91	11.50	56.0
Distance of mother from farthest child	10.91	14.64	54.0

Notes: *p < .05
***p < .001

desired. In addition, following the intervention in the treatment group, there is a significant reduction in scatteredness between the mother and the child farthest from her or the one closest to her, as compared with the control group. We found that the more children in the family, the greater the distance between each parent and the children. Correlations were found between the number of children and the distance between the mother and children ($r = .54$; $p < .01$), and between the father and children ($r = .73$; $p < .001$).

Another concept reflected in KFST is that of family hierarchy (Ecklad and Vandvik, 1992). In the hierarchical family, the subject places the parents above the children, and in the nonhierarchical family, the subject places the parents parallel to or below the children (see Figure 11.4).

No significant differences were found using the chi-square test between the groups, before or after the intervention.

To sum up, as we had hypothesized, more change appeared in the experimental group than in the control group in the area of family structure after completing the intervention, albeit only in two dimensions out of ten. Some possible explanations for these results will be discussed later in the chapter.

Additional Findings

We shall present here findings between the dependent variables in family functioning and family structure. Table 11.7 shows the correlations between dimensions of family structure and family functioning for both men and women.

Among women, we found a high correlation in the distance between the couple and the following dimensions of family functioning: problem solving, roles, affective involvement, and affective responsiveness. Among men, we found significant correlations in the distance between the couple and their extended families and the following dimensions of family functioning: problem solving, affective involvement, and affective responsiveness (see Table 11.7). The greater the distance between the couple and the extended family, the poorer the men's functioning.

FIGURE 11.4. Examples of Hierarchical and Nonhierarchical Families

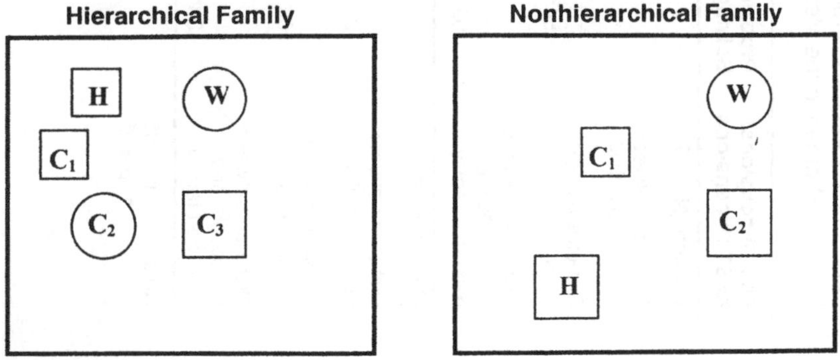

TABLE 11.7. Pearson Correlation Between Dimensions of Family Structure and Dimensions of Family Functioning Among Men and Women in the Measurement, Before Treatment Intervention

FAD Dimensions: KFST Dimensions	Problem Solving	Communication	Roles	Affective Responsiveness	Affective Involvement	Control	General Functioning
Women (N = 25)							
Distance between mother and child	.13	-.17	-.09	-.27	-.01	-.12	-.07
Distance between the spouses	.54**	.25	.54**	.41*	.41*	.18	.24
Distance between the couple and extended family	-.02	.10	-.04	-.01	-.33*	.29	-.01
Men (N = 24)							
Distance between father and child	.31	-.05	.11	-.11	.17	.01	.06
Distance between the spouses	.06	.19	.20	-.23	.09	.17	-.10
Distance between the couple and extended family	.38*	.02	.19	.36*	.46*	.34*	-.10

Notes: * $p < .05$
** $p < .01$

Summary and Conclusions of the Quantitative Analysis

Our goal in this research was to evaluate the effectiveness of the project's interventions with FED, as measured by both family functioning and family structure. Our sample was divided into two groups. One was the experimental group, which participated in ten therapeutic sessions. The second was the control group, which was not involved in treatment sessions. Both groups filled out questionnaires before the beginning of the intervention, as well as at the end of the project (see Table 11.8).

Family functioning was found to be relatively low before the project began. The intervention resulted in better family functioning in the dimensions of problem solving and affective involvement, as well as improvement in the husbands' "behavior control." These changes can be understood on various levels. The issue of problem-solving skills was one of the major concerns during treatment in dealing with problems raised by FED. The family members were encouraged to help themselves in their efforts to solve their difficulties. Taking care of one another and showing an interest in one another's values contributed to increasing affection and involvement among family members.

A great deal of attention was given by FED to their children, which resulted in the improvement in fathers' behavior control, as measured by the Family Assessment Device, and in an improved relationship between the mothers and their children, as measured by KFST. It is important to indicate that the mothers in FED were more dominant and more stable, with a better score in general functioning than the fathers. It can be assumed that a longer intervention might also result in the father's improved functioning, as well as an improvement in the functioning of the couple's subsystem. Marital changes are usually slower and require more than ten intervention sessions. Furthermore, it would seem that most of the families could not focus on marital issues before dealing with problems of their daily existence, such as financial hardships and problems between children and parents. Therefore, it is strongly recommended to have ten additional therapy sessions, following a short period of absorption and reflection. This is true even when relating to the subjective evaluation of the families, and when case managers consider the interventions to be helpful and meaningful.

TABLE 11.8. Summary of the Major Findings of the Quantitative Analysis

Variables Tested	Hypothesis	Instrument	Major Findings
Family Functioning	Following treatment intervention, there will be an improvement in the family functioning, as measured before treatment. No differences between measurements "before" and "after" in the control group.	FAD	Improvements were found in the following dimensions: (1) Problem solving (2) Affective involvement (3) Behavior control No major differences found between genders except for general functioning, where women reported better functioning than men.
Family Structure	There will be a change in the family structure between the measurements "before" and "after" the intervention. No change will be observed in the control group.	KFST	Change was found in the following dimensions: (1) Distance between the couple and the extended family (2) Distance between the mother and the children No gender differences were found in relation to hierarchical or nonhierarchical position.

It is also important to indicate the limitations of this project's findings. One major limitation can be attributed to the small sample size of both our treatment and control groups. Another problem was the use of instruments that were primarily standardized to a higher-level socioeconomic population. Our subjects had difficulties in reading and writing, low frustration tolerance, and low concentration ability. To overcome some of these problems, we read the questionnaires to our subjects, used cards, and made some changes in the vocabulary. However, we encountered numerous difficulties in our attempts to elicit responses to the KFST, with reactions of family members ranging from inattention to quarrels. In the future, we recommend that the entire family, not only the spouses, undergo the KFST. Finally, it is important to note that standardized instruments are often not sensitive enough to measure changes occurring after ten sessions.

THE SUBJECTIVE EVALUATION

Subjective evaluation can also be described as clinical evaluation. We refer to three different reports, given by (1) the family, during the last meeting (Session #10); (2) the case manager, in a summary written at the end of the project; and (3) the family therapist, during a postproject interview. The reports refer to changes that occurred within the family and between the family and external systems. They are based on the contract signed with the family and are related to the specific goals of each family. Also taken into account is the degree of satisfaction the family gained from the treatment. A question may be asked regarding this last point. Can we consider a level of satisfaction as an indicator of success even if there are no visible signs of change? Our answer is yes. We decided to take into account the degree of satisfaction based on the assumption that if the family had a positive experience in the treatment process, it might provide motivation to continue with treatment. No doubt, the intervention in this project was brief in view of the gravity of the problems faced by each family. However, it is our belief and evaluation that this positive experience generated the necessary confidence among family members that they can be helped and that they can cope with treatment intervention (Bandura, 1977).

The S. Family

The Family

The family feels that there is a better atmosphere and less tension at home. The couple has returned to sleeping together and can now share their difficulties. Mrs. S. is able to stand up to her husband's anger without feeling threatened. As reported by Mrs. S., Mr. S. is willing, for the first time in his life, to go out to work. Mr. S. feels more appreciative of his wife and notes that she is taking better care of her appearance. She initiates affection, provides him with security, and cares for him.

The Social Worker

The couple was able to take upon themselves various tasks, including difficult ones, even during treatment sessions. They have begun to speak directly to each other about intimate feelings. As a result of these changes, the wife has started to take better care of herself, invest more in the home, and look for a job. The couple is now attempting to take responsibility for paying back their debts, functioning better as parents, and attending to their marital conflicts.

The Family Therapist

Changes in communication skills are evident. The spouses can look at and address each other directly. Mrs. S. is less frightened of her husband. There is a change in the family balance in that Mrs. S. is no longer the only "good one" who wants her husband to go to work, while he refuses. The treatment seems to have clarified for them how she had neither encouraged nor enabled him to go out to work. The couple has returned to sleeping together, and Mrs. S. is now taking better care of herself and her home, while also thinking about looking for a job. The couple has begun to understand what is meant by personal responsibility and has made an attempt at paying their debts by asking for unification of their files. The request was filed in court several times and was finally granted. (However, the couple failed in utilizing the training they had received in preparing their daughter for surgery.)

The Z. Family

The Family

Mr. Z. says that the treatment helped him to "get one or two wheels out of the mud, but not the entire wagon, and there is still a long way to go." Mr. Z. claims that he was successful in getting his daughter K. back to school by talking to her and making her certain promises. He did this by himself, without the help of Mrs. Z. Mr. Z. asserts that, in his opinion, and in light of what was said during treatment, Mrs. Z. should get out of their children's lives and let them grow. Mrs. Z. states that she did not receive any help, that the Department of Social Services is useless, and that no one ever helps there. Furthermore, their son A. should be put in an institution, and nobody cares. (According to tests A. underwent, he should not leave the home; other forms of more suitable arrangements were suggested, but all were rejected by the family.)

The Social Worker

Mr. Z. has become somewhat stronger as head of the family, partly as a result of the change in the couple's balance. Signs of a beginning in communication between the spouses can be observed, such as the way in which they approach the DSS and directly present their problems. K. has returned to school after a long absence due to the collaborative efforts of many systems, including the parents, the school, the special education teacher, and the truant officer.

The Family Therapist

K., who was out of school for several months, was able to return to school. R., the older daughter, got married and began the process of separation from her family, even though it was very difficult for the parents. There are still problems with two or three children, but the father, who gained strength through therapy, began communicating directly with the children and supporting them, while setting boundaries between the parental subsystem and that of the children. A decrease in Mrs. Z.'s destructive functioning has been observed, and she has returned to doing her household chores.

The L. Family

The Family

Both the couple and their children report that there have been fewer quarrels between the spouses and that Mrs. L. screams and curses less. Mr. L. stated that "she screams approximately two hours a day now, instead of twelve hours," and that he forgives her. Both spouses indicate that they speak more with each other and that they are now able "to cry with each other." Despite Mrs. L.'s fear of remaining alone, she is ready to see Mr. L. go for alcohol addiction treatment and is even happy about it. Mr. L. is very interested in the treatment and points out that he and Mrs. L. have a much better relationship now. The children state that they are happy to hear the parents talk about weaning (detoxification) treatment. Furthermore, they report that in addition to the change in the relationship between the parents, their own relationship with the parents has improved. They are now able to understand the pain that caused their mother to cry and their father to drink, something that they had not been aware of before the treatment. Everyone at home is now more open about stating his or her opinion and saying what hurt him or her in the past. All point to the fact that G., one of the children, decided to remain at home instead of going to the boarding school, which she had previously considered because of conflict with her mother. All express regret about the treatment being over.

The Social Worker

The social worker says that she was afraid of Mrs. L. returning for hospitalization, but when this did not happen, it was an achievement in itself. In addition, the couple has started talking and listening to each other, even looking at each other rather than constantly hitting and cursing. The family has begun to discuss treating Mr. L.'s alcoholism. The elder daughters have become less involved in their parents' quarrels and feel less responsible for their parents' life. G. has made an independent choice to remain at home and has restored her relationship with her mother.

The Family Therapist

Some boundaries and family organization have been achieved in the family. The girls no longer assume responsibility for their parents' life. G. is not leaving home, and the parents have some support and are seeming to cope successfully with their daughter I. and her acting out. I. is being raised by her aunt and comes to her parents' home only for visits. On the communication level, family members now recognize their part in the conflicts, which seem to have calmed down, and there is more communication between the parents and the children. Mr. L. has agreed to go for alcohol abuse treatment.

The E. Family

The Family

Mrs. E. states that in these conversations, she was able to open her heart for the first time without the fear that Mr. E. would beat her, adding that her husband allowed her to do so. Mr. E. says that nothing has changed, but that he appreciates how the social worker has tried to help him. He also mentions his willingness to go back to work. Both spouses remark that they anticipated the therapeutic meetings and felt the readiness of others to help them. They appreciate the work done with the educational system; nonetheless, they are disappointed that the system did not provide the help they needed.

The Social Worker

The family has begun "opening windows," and its members have stopped pretending that they have no problems. They have started talking about existing problems between the spouses. It appears that some trust has been developing between the family, the social worker, the family therapist, and other Department of Social Services personnel.

The Family Therapist

The treatment has allowed the spouses to release some of their anger toward society and, to a very limited extent, to touch on their problems as a couple, while reflecting on past issues. They have started talking with their daughter P., allowing her to choose which school to go to, and have supported her decision in spite of their different views. A great deal of effort has been invested in dealing with the daughter's educational system to help her get back into a learning framework.

The N. Family

The Family

The family claims that nothing has changed, but that they are willing to continue the meetings. Mr. N. remarks that even if he does find work, he will ask the boss to allow him to meet with the team, since the possibility to express himself makes him feel better. Mrs. N. says that she would also join the sessions because, similar to her husband, she feels the need to express herself. At the end of the meeting, the family asked to take a picture of the team.

The Social Worker

There is evidence of a little more understanding and communication, although Mrs. N. does not seem to feel it. Mr. N. seems able to control himself better and has made an effort to find work, although so far he has been unsuccessful.

The Family Therapist

The structure of the present treatment has been different from that of past interventions. This is the first time that they have had joint family therapy rather than the individual treatments, given previously only to Mrs. N. The treatment provided a place to express their ideas, their needs, and their wishes. During treatment, Mr. N. was given a great deal of support; however, the team emphasized restraining Mr. N.'s aggression toward his wife and toward social institutions. All meetings reflected a continuous decrease in his violence against Mrs. N. He was accompanied on his job hunting in an attempt to help him cope with his characteristic fears, most specifically, his own violent tendencies. Mr. N.'s role as a parent has also been strengthened through treatment.

The G. Family

The Family

Following a discussion regarding the home, the G.s cleaned their house; it now looks tidier and the kids have stopped drawing on walls. Mrs. G. has gone to visit her mother, with Mr. G.'s approval and encouragement. She gained a great deal of strength from this visit. Although it was very difficult for the parents to accept the fact that A. needs special education training, they have helped him to obtain the appropriate assistance.

The Social Worker

The social worker believes that this family needs to be coached on a variety of small, everyday matters to maintain the changes that have been achieved by the family during treatment, such as setting boundaries for the children.

The Family Therapist

This is a very impoverished family. The father seems to be slightly retarded, and the mother has a history of psychiatric treatments. The intervention has been targeted on a very concrete level. The most notable change has been in establishing clearer boundaries for the children, as expressed in stopping them from drawing on walls. A., their son, has begun doing some work with a special education training teacher, with Mrs. G.'s approval. They have not placed their youngest daughter in a nursery school, in spite of the effort made to convince them to do so.

The LK. Family

The Family

The family dropped out of treatment after five sessions.

The Social Worker

Therapy ended after five sessions. Mrs. LK. wanted very much to continue with the treatment for herself, but that would have reinforced the family's pattern, in which Mr. LK. leaves all responsibilities to his wife.

The Family Therapist

Therapy ended after five sessions since the family members were not at home when the therapeutic team arrived. Nevertheless, some changes did occur at the very beginning of treatment. Mr. LK. returned to work. He bought a truck and worked in moving goods and fishing. K., who had been living with his grandparents, came back to live with his parents. His behavior in school improved, and he started concentrating on his studies. Mrs. LK. asked to continue the treatment for herself, but it was decided not to do so as part of the FED project. About one month later, Mrs. LK. applied again for help to the Department of Social Services. The social worker insisted on meeting with the entire family, and the family agreed.

The SA. Family

The Family

Mr. and Mrs. SA. indicate that they are more aware now of their part in what happens at home and of the pain both of them have caused each other. They have learned to listen and to relate to each other with more understanding, realizing that quite often anger is the result of weakness and stress. They want to continue living together because they love each other. They definitely want things to be different, to be better. They appreciate the treatment sessions, saying, "It's not like being with the guys from the neighborhood . . ." Mr. SA. has begun to understand the influence of drinking and to consider joining a rehabilitation program.

The Social Worker

The social worker points out the family's participation at all the meetings. It seems that the couple has hope and is aware of the possibility for help. Following treatment, they have a higher awareness of the part that each of them has contributed to family quarrels.

They have begun communicating directly with each other and with more respect. They have touched on the subject of weaning treatment, but are still at the very beginning of the process. Mr. SA. realizes that he has to look for different work with higher income potential.

The Family Therapist

The change can be observed on the couple level. Each one of the spouses has become aware of his or her part in creating conflict. Mrs. SA. has learned to identify her ways of weakening Mr. SA. and how to let him reenter the family. Mr. SA., in turn, has tried to help his wife take care of the children. There seems to be some movement toward organizing financial issues, including Mr. SA.'s looking for a new job to increase the family income. Overall, the couple appears to have benefited from the therapeutic dialogue.

The A. Family

The Family

The family expresses satisfaction from the change in parenting and feels that cooperation between the spouses has contributed to the children's well-being. The family notes that they listen to one another more at home. Mr. A. feels that he is more involved in planning things at home and is willing to assume more responsibility for the children and his wife.

The Social Worker

As a result of treatment, there is a stronger relationship between the father and the children. The father has taken on more responsibilities. He now feels more personally involved with each family member and has been celebrating the children's birthdays. The couple has learned to give more thought to the children's emotions. The oldest son will return home at the end of the school year, after living with his grandparents. However, it seems that the new responsibilities have somewhat overwhelmed Mr. A., and he has started acting out.

The Family Therapist

Treatment has been focused on the parental level, in spite of existing spousal problems. The parents have learned how to work as a team and have undertaken the responsibility of role division. Throughout the process, there has been noticeable role flexibility, for example, Mr. A. starting to help with the cooking. Reports from school have revealed the children's progress, likely due to the father's new involvement in the children's education. However, the stress of the new functioning seems to have threatened him, and as a result, he committed burglary. During the weeks he spent in jail, his wife functioned well, something he could not ignore, and he even complemented her on it. Toward the end of the treatment, Mr. A. expressed his willingness to go to weaning treatment and to attend a retraining program in gardening or to become a barber.

The B. Family

The Family

Mrs. B. feels that she has changed, saying, "Before you came, I was dead. Now I am beginning to live." She assumes more responsibility around the house. Mr. B. remarks that his wife looks better now and is paying more attention to the house. As a result, he too is helping more around the house, as well as going out to work. For the last session, the family prepared a heart-shaped cake together; the father bought the ingredients and the wife baked the cake.

The Social Worker

Some communication lines have opened up between husband and wife. The wife is more open and has begun talking about problems, while the husband has begun working.

The Family Therapist

The family therapist was changed after three meetings. This must have had some impact on the process, which was short and not too rewarding. It was difficult to reach a focused working contract with the family, yet it seems that a positive result of the treatment process is that Mr. B. has started to work, in spite of his illness. Mrs. B. has started functioning better at home despite her CVA. She has also begun thinking about sending her daughter to kindergarten. The couple opened up to each other, started discussing their problems, with Mrs. B. feeling less inhibited. At the last session, the family prepared a heart-shaped cake with very touching words for the team.

The AD. Family

The Family

Mr. AD. is willing to go for weaning treatment. Mrs. AD. has indicated that she has gained more strength and is now looking for further changes, since she is not ready to continue with things as they are today. Mr. AD. requests that she not ignore the good things they have accomplished together. They both stated that they are sorry the children were not present at the therapeutic meetings, as they feel they have gained a great deal from them.

The Social Worker

There is significant change at the level of parent-child relationships. N. has developed a positive point of view toward his parents, which, in turn, has enabled him to regain his place as a child, rather than a parental child. The couple has learned how to sit and talk to each other, not only about immediate problems, but also about thoughts and feelings, as well as how to accept each other's faults and good points. They have gained strength in coping with very hard times.

The Family Therapist

As a result of treatment, clearer boundaries have been established between the parents and their children. The parents have learned to separate the children, especially the older one, N., who became a parental child as soon as there was a problem between the parents. Consequently, N. has gone back to school. Mrs. AD. is better than her husband at setting clear-cut boundaries, but he joins her from time to time. Because of the regular therapeutic sessions, the DSS has been able to gain more accurate information on the family's economic difficulties and heavy debts and to search for possible remedies for this situation. Mr. AD. has realized that he cannot stop his drug addiction by himself and has started looking for weaning programs being developed in France. His wife has encouraged him to join the weaning program, indicating that she is not willing to return to live together with Mr. AD. while he is still on drugs. She has stopped accepting drug-addicted friends into their home so that the children do not see them taking drugs. Despite being defined as a mental health patient, she displays considerable strength in daily functioning.

The ES. Family

The Family

The husband notes that he feels less isolated following the meetings. He can now talk about various topics. His wife indicates that she has learned to do many things for the family. Today, she knows how to define her expectations of her husband, namely, that he should play with the children. During the last meeting, family members brought various personal belongings that they wanted to share with the team.

The Social Worker

Following treatment, the family has been able to sit together as a family for the first time. As a result of the treatment, they have begun to take better care of the house and the children and to be involved in the children's education.

The Family Therapist

Following treatment, members of the family have begun talking to one another, including the father, for the first time. Previously, he had remained isolated, while his wife gathered her children around her. As a result of the treatment, the father has indicated his willingness to change the way in which he and his wife communicate. He now recognizes his weaknesses at home, both as a man and as a father. This openness has been achieved despite the family's initial resistance to participating in the project. They finally decided to take part in the project, but only because they thought it would bring them economic compensation.

The F. Family

The Family

(Only the wife and the children participated.) Following treatment, Mrs. F. feels much stronger and less alone. She has learned how to play with the children and how to discipline them, as well as how to enjoy herself. Now, the children keep much busier and quarrel less. They have better control of themselves, even regarding bed-wetting. At the end of treatment, the children gave the team members drawings and a letter saying, "We want you," and the mother requested further conversations.

The Social Worker

The mother has gained strength, showing more authority in disciplining her children, and is getting some collaboration in return. She has more control over what happens at home between her and the children and between her and her husband. Mr. F. does not physically or verbally abuse her in front of the children. The children are more organized because they experience clearer boundaries and discipline. They are also less violent toward one another. Their self-image has improved, and they show more restraint and confidence.

The Family Therapist

The family therapist was changed after three meetings. The father stopped coming to treatment. He is an alcoholic, wandering around all day, without any responsibilities at home. It was decided not to stop treatment but rather to give Mrs. F. the support and tools to cope with the children alone. As a result, she has started playing more with the children and setting boundaries. Although her husband has been beating her for a long time, she never complained to the police, but now, after being involved in treatment, she has found the courage to file a complaint with the police. She feels stronger as a woman and as a mother. She has stopped sleeping with the children and has developed a good relationship with their school.

The M. Family

The Family

Role division has been initiated so that the children help more, each one doing something at home. Likewise, the parents pay more attention to the children. At the end of treatment, the children made drawings and wrote farewell letters saying, "It's a pity you are leaving."

The Social Worker

No report.

The Family Therapist

Most work has been done on the parental level, focusing on reinforcing the parents as a team, dividing the responsibilities at home, and relating in a different manner to the children.

The C. Family

Treatment was stopped after four sessions, as it became apparent that to achieve any progress whatsoever with this family, multiprofessional teamwork would have to be applied. The social worker was unable to organize such a meeting; meanwhile, contact with the family was interrupted.

The D. Family

The family was not classified as FED. They had a very sick child around whom all their problems were centered. The father refused to cooperate right from the beginning, while the mother, afraid that her position as a mother might be compromised, declined any further contact.

The K. Family

The Family

No summary was reported. The family made the effort to arrive at the Haifa Center for Family Therapy for live supervision by the family therapist. This step indicated family members' interest and readiness to invest in the treatment.

The Social Worker

No report.

The Family Therapist

As a result of treatment, boundaries have been defined between the role of the parents and the role of the grandparents. An understanding was reached that the children would not go to live with the grandparents. However, they could not stay at home permanently either because the mother was unable to stop herself from beating and abusing them. Consequently, a permanent schedule was established that divided the children's time between the parents and the grandparents. This has brought some order to the children's lives and avoided confusion. During treatment, boundaries were established between parents and children. The daughter was released from the role of the parental child. Toward the end of treatment, the mother was able to show more control and restraint. The parents have invested more effort in their contact with the children, allowing the children more separation and the beginning of some individualization. During treatment, Mr. K. also began to work.

SUMMARY

Table 11.9 summarizes the clinical changes as observed by the families, social workers (case managers), and family therapists. These changes are defined as follows:

1. *Change in the couple's communication:* any improvement in the ability of the couple to talk things over, to listen, to speak instead of using violence, to relate to the spouse's difficulties, to ask for help directly, to pay compliments, and so forth.
2. *Change in family/couple functioning:* a change in the family balance, as reflected in setting boundaries, becoming better organized, going out to work, assuming responsibilities, sleeping together again, and so on.
3. *Change in parenting:* any change in the parental functioning toward the children, such as setting boundaries, supporting or playing with the children.
4. *Change on the individual level:* behavioral or cognitive change in at least one member of the family, as manifested in his or her attempts to be treated for alcoholism or drug abuse, to work, to assume the role of parent or child in a more functional way, and so on.
5. *Satisfaction with treatment:* voiced verbally or nonverbally, for example, the willingness to be photographed with the team, baking a cake, preparing a drawing, and so forth.

In our summary, we did not refer to the extent of the change because we had not asked family members, the social worker, or the therapist to rate the changes separately on a scale. Moreover, our basic inclination before starting the intervention treatment with the FED was not to expect more than minimal movement in each family. As evident in a review of the relevant literature, other attempts in working with multiproblem families have shown that little change can be expected. The number of problems and their chronicity does not allow for dramatic change. Expecting major changes can only lead to frustration. We emphasized this point and prepared our workers in this direction. However, even with this approach in mind, we have seen changes taking place among our families in various areas. These changes have been identified by more than one

TABLE 11.9 Summary of Clinical Evaluation by Family/Social Worker/Family Therapist

Family	Change in Couple Communication	Change in Family/ Couple Functioning	Change in Parenthood	Individual Change	Satisfaction from Treatment
S.	x * +	x * +		x * +	x * +
Z.	*	x *	x +	+	x * +
L.	x * +	x * +	x * +	x * +	x * +
E.	+	x +			
N.	* +			* +	x
G.			x +		x *
LK.				+	+
SA.	x * +	x * +		x * +	x * +
A.	x	x	x * +		
B.	x * +	x * +		x * +	x * +
AD.	*	*	* +	x * +	x
ES.		x *	x * +	+	x +
F.			* +	* +	* +
M.(2)			* +	*	
C.(1)					
D.(1)					
K.(3)		+	+		

x = Change reported by the family.
* = Change reported by the social worker.
+ = Change reported by the family therapist.
(1) = Family stopped treatment—no evaluation.
(2) = Evaluation by social worker is missing.

source, namely, the family, social worker, or family therapist, or even by all three evaluators.

Table 11.9 reveals that, with the exception of the two families in which treatment was interrupted, each family underwent at least two changes, and usually more. This evaluation may raise once more the dilemma of the discrepancy between the clinical, subjective evaluation and the use of objective instruments. We shall save the reader from this debate and conclude with our experience, since we used both a quantitative research design, including objective and subjective tools, and a qualitative study to explore the therapeutic process. We incorporated some of the qualitative findings that were related to the intervention process in Chapters 6 and 7 on the "toolbox," thus presenting some of the findings from our analysis regarding the content of our interventions. In this chapter, we presented the quantitative findings and ended with the subjective evaluation. Using these three methods, namely, qualitative, quantitative, and subjective evaluation, we have been able to achieve much more than by a single research method alone. For one thing, they complement each other. Second, they may serve to validate some of the resultant changes. Finally, it seems that in working with FED, by adapting expectations for minimal intervention goals, we may be able to avoid worker and family burnout in these cases.

Our findings show that the FED taking part in the project have achieved a great deal during the ten treatment sessions. Although measured globally, the most meaningful finding is, no doubt, the new positive experience with treatment, as clearly indicated by almost all the families in our project. The positive experience for families is that treatment may lead to certain changes; it certainly serves as a basis for hope and the possibility of continued progress.

PART VI: FUTURE PERSPECTIVES

Chapter 12

Considerations and Attempts for Hope

In summary, we raise several questions. In terms of our main interest, which was working with families in extreme distress, could, and should, poor and distressed families be helped? How should they be helped? What have we done so far? Have we helped to relieve FED of their distress? Finally, where do we go from here? Can we suggest some strategic views? What do we suggest for FED in the future? What can be done to prevent families from becoming distressed? We shall attempt to address these questions in this final chapter.

Our point of departure, inasmuch as it may sound fatalistic, is the suggestion that poverty is a phenomenon that will be with us for a long time. We end a century that began with wars and starvation, with poverty and distress, but then raised some hope for social changes that might bring more families a measure of comfort and well-being. No doubt, we have come a long way, but, unfortunately, we enter a new century facing the possibility of even more dangerous wars and a greater number of poor people.

Many of our society's resources are still allocated to "war building." Diplomatic exercises are performed to avoid war and destruction. Huge efforts are invested in developing increasingly sophisticated technology used for military and other purposes. This, in turn, widens the gap of social stratification and creates more poor and distressed families. Models are generated for decreasing tension and conflict. We learn to negotiate, to mediate, to solve problems in a diplomatic manner.

Now it is our responsibility to prepare a similar set of "diplomatic" solutions for the social ills caused by this relentless process that would be used as tools in the "war against poverty." As we progress toward the twenty-first century, building a healthier society becomes our greatest challenge. However, we see that maintaining a welfare state has become more complex and is often criticized by economists and other policymakers. Consequently, fewer resources are made available to develop programs for helping FED. This brings us to our first question: Should poor families be helped, even though we can foresee that their problems will persist? Let us try to answer this question by looking at the case of the S. family.*

Several years after completing the project, one of the writers taught a course on families in extreme distress, where she met a student who was doing her field training at the Department of Social Services, which had taken part in the project. During a discussion, the student shared with the class an example from the S. family in our project. In the course of her work, the student had met with Mrs. S., who was working as a volunteer at the Department of Social Services helping the staff with interventions with FED. Once a month, she also made an anonymous donation to help any desperate family in need. Mrs. S. told the student that her family, too, had been in a desperate situation, but ever since they were chosen to take part in a therapeutic project, things had changed. Her husband, who had always invested a great deal of effort to support his family, was encouraged to go for alcohol abuse treatment. The treatment was successful, to a great extent because of the family's support. Following treatment, he had more confidence to go out and find a new job. This helped to improve their financial situation to the point that they decided to venture into private business and opened a fruit and vegetable store. Today, they feel that they can make a contribution to society, just as they were once helped.

No doubt, the case of the S. family supported Dewey's (1933) idea that people can change, grow, and develop. When society invests in programs aimed at developing people, it can usually expect some return from those who benefit as a result of these programs. This philosophy is what has guided society in its efforts to create programs for the poor. In keeping with Dewey's perspective, we also believe that if society were not to help the poor, the end result would be a rise in delinquency, violence, drug abuse, and sickness that would affect the

*The case was described in detail in Sharlin, Shamai, and Gilad-Smolinsky (1994).

entire society, including those considered fit. There is, therefore, sufficient justification supporting the need to work with FED. This brings us to our next question: How do we do it?

We have learned from our project that FED can and should be helped. We even dare to say that there are no unmotivated clients, but rather unmotivated, threatened social workers and family therapists who are afraid to enter the clients' desperate world and learn their language and culture. Such fears often create in social workers and family therapists feelings of hopelessness and helplessness, similar to those of the FED clients themselves. We refer to this phenomenon as a coalition of despair. This coalition can be transformed into a coalition of hope by utilizing the knowledge acquired about these families. In fact, a better understanding of the FED problem, along with the know-how in developing the skills and techniques necessary for therapeutic intervention, may be the only resources available for helping FED to resolve their distress predicament, in view of the negligible financial assistance provided by the government.

Let us summarize what we have learned from our project:

1. FED can be detected early by examining nine different categories: poverty, housing, health, couple functioning, parental functioning, children, substance abuse, antisocial behavior, and support systems. Furthermore, each of these categories can be measured, studied, and observed. Once detected, clinical decision making can take place with the clients, the family, and the community.
2. We have learned the importance of seeing the clients in their own home environments. This was mainly done to avoid having to organize their visits to the Department of Social Services, since these chronically disorganized families would most likely not stay on schedule. This also helped to increase the clients' trust in their therapists' deep desire to help the family. It also gave the team an opportunity to observe the clients in their everyday milieu.
3. The use of a therapeutic team rather than one social worker or family therapist prevented the team from entering into a coalition of despair with the family. This approach appeared to be

more expensive at the beginning, but in the long run, it was more effective and increased accountability.

4. In planning structured and focused interventions, it became clear that the dialogue with the family was essential in defining the problems and the therapeutic goals that were relevant to the family, as well as a way to achieve these goals.
5. Developing and using a "toolbox," which includes a repertoire of various techniques, can help the team to fit the appropriate technique to the specific family problem. Furthermore, having possible answers and solutions for unforeseen problems raises the team's professional confidence.

There is a wealth of knowledge that can be used in working with FED. It can be implemented by a social worker or a family therapist when working with one or more families or by an agency with a group of social workers involved in a project. Furthermore, cooperation among several agencies can be greatly enhanced by this knowledge and experience in their attempt to take up the challenge of working with FED. This can involve policy intervention, such as creating a special center for FED, or even social action toward developing a welfare policy (see Figure 12.1). These possibilities might seem more in the realm of Utopian dreams, since reality allows only their modest implementation. Nevertheless, past experience teaches us that some principles, perspectives, concepts, strategies, and techniques can be utilized in answering questions about intervention with FED and in planning future directions for intervention with this population.

INTERVENTION

The main question about future intervention with FED refers to the principles that will guide the intervention. Will it provide a context in which FED are taught how to acquire middle-class values and culture? Will it be a process through which FED will search for alternatives for solving their difficulties? Will it be a process that will demarginalize them? It seems to us that all of these questions are the focus of the intervention and should be approached according to the desire of each family. Therefore, we suggest two guiding

FIGURE 12.1. The Various Systems for Intervention with FED

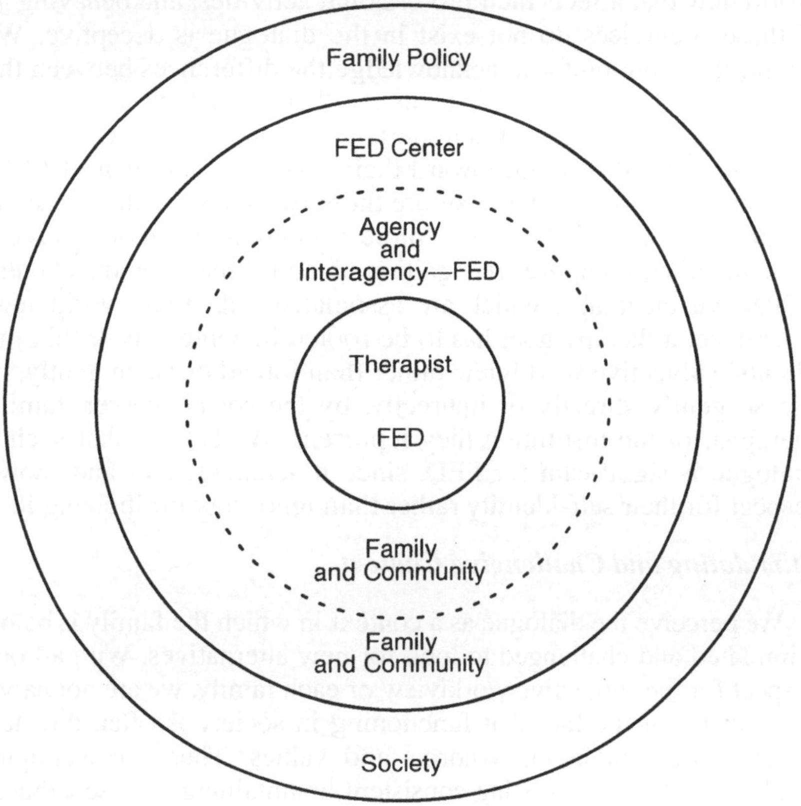

principles for the intervention: (1) dialogue and (2) a stimulating and challenging context.

Dialogue

A dialogue means providing an equal place for therapists and families to express their ideas and feelings. It means that the decision about whether to join the intervention, specific goals of the intervention, and individual tasks within the intervention are negotiable and created by the dialogue between the participants. Dialogue also means acknowledging that social workers and family therapists bring their own prejudices to the dialogue, including personal values, culture, and ideology. Such prejudices create a worldview that affects their professional activities, and behaving as if these prejudices do not exist in the dialogue is deceptive. We would therefore prefer to acknowledge the differences between the worldview of the therapeutic team and that of the family.

To create a dialogue, it is important for the practitioners to hold an open-minded position toward their own view and that of FED. This means being ready to explore these two views without assuming that one view is "better," "more accurate," or "more correct" than the other. It requires recognition of, and respect for, the clients' subjective meanings, which are associated with their worldview. Therefore, a therapy goal has to be rooted in some way within the clients' subjective worldview rather than forced on them gently, or not so gently, directly or indirectly, by the social worker, family therapist, or the institution they represent. We believe that such a dialogue is significant for FED, since it acknowledges and shows respect for their self-identity rather than ignoring or criticizing it.

Stimulating and Challenging Context

We perceive the dialogue as a context in which the family is being stimulated and challenged to look for new alternatives. With all our respect for the subjective worldview of each family, we are not naive or unaware of the fact that functioning in society is often directed according to middle-class norms and values. Thus, for example, holding a job requires being consistent, maintaining time schedules, and overcoming frustrations. Succeeding in school also requires consistency, concentration, and the ability to cope with frustrations. Without success in school, the probability of getting an interesting and well-paid job is reduced. It is, therefore, the role of the therapeutic team to challenge FED to find channels through which they can integrate their subjective worldview with the norms that are often accepted by the wider, middle-class society. It is, however, not our intention to suggest that they abandon their traditional ethnic values, customs, and norms.

The balance between challenging the family and creating a respectful dialogue seems to us the art and the core of future interventions with FED. Such a balance becomes even more crucial, if not precarious, when therapy with FED is required by law, such as in cases of child abuse. The ability to create a dialogue with the family in which hierarchy and power do not dictate the goals and form of therapy is a major task for those who work with FED.

Many family therapists avoid being labeled as agents of "social institutions" and thus leave public service in favor of private practice, while criticizing workers in social agencies who try to keep an almost impossible balance between "nonhierarchical" intervention and dialogue. As social workers and family therapists, we believe that intervention with FED is possible almost exclusively in public services. We also believe in the role of society to defend any human being in cases of abuse, and we strongly believe that FED can create a warm context for raising children, even if they fail in some other functioning goals. Therefore, it is the art of working with FED and the commitment of these social workers and family therapists that determines the success of moving between dialogue and intervention, recognizing hierarchy while respecting the client, and relating to the power in an ethical and moral way. Unfortunately, this is complicated and often cannot be done without losing the balance, but this complexity seems to be the nature of intervention with FED and the challenge of working with this population.

PERSPECTIVE OF INTERVENTION

Intervention with FED has to be multilevel and must take into account individuals and families, community, and society at large. It is important to indicate that working on the different levels does not require one team. It is possible to create teams that focus and develop knowledge and skills to intervene on each level.

We view society's cultural level as the basis for allowing intervention with FED. It is necessary that society recognize the existence of FED instead of ignoring the phenomenon. The ability of society to accept its responsibility for the development of FED, as well as its responsibility to demarginalize these families, allows professionals to find ways of joining with this population. Such an attitude provides room for cultural, ethnic, and gender diversity, for different forms of families, such as single-parent families, and for the subjective meanings that different families give to their experience in society.

This kind of societal attitude, however, does not just suddenly "appear." It requires intensive involvement with policymakers, the media, and the educational system. It calls for social action—an "old," yet relevant, task of social workers and other professionals with a social view. It requires the development of a family policy, which we shall discuss briefly later on. Intervention with families has to be sensitive to the different forms of families created by modern society. Maintaining an understanding of traditional family values causes strain within many families, especially in single-parent families, which are often affected by women's inequality in society, making it necessary to deal with gender issues as well.

Based on our experience, we strongly believe in the ability of FED to join and use more than just a channel for concrete financial help. We found desperate families that were looking for someone who would give them some hope. It was the dialogue with respectful listening that affected their self-esteem and increased their self-respect. We think that family intervention with FED has to be integrative and flexible. It should use as many techniques as possible, without being "loyal" to any one specific set of techniques. It calls for a large toolbox that allows the therapist to respect the specific needs and culture of each family. It requires the skills to move between the subsystems within the family and to be aware if further interventions are needed on an individual level.

Similar to Minuchin (1974), we perceive the parents, or parent, as the leaders of the family and believe that through effective dialogue, they will be empowered and able to open new alternatives for the family, themselves, and their children. We believe that working with the family can help to create a nurturing context for the adults and the children. Although we used extended families in only a few cases in our project, we found that their inclusion in therapy may be very helpful to the nuclear families. This option has to be investigated and, if possible, used as a support system in stressful situations.

The community can also contribute a lot to the development of a nurturing context. We suggest implementation of the following:

1. Health services with sensitivity to cultural, ethnic, and gender diversity, as well as to the subjective worldview of each fam-

ily. Most of these services exist, but require special training for their staff to develop such sensitivity skills.

2. Day and/or afternoon care for children that will operate until late afternoons and thus help working parents to finish their working hours, rest, and then be able to provide a warm and nurturing context for their children. This might reduce the tendency to remove children from the parental home to institutions or foster homes.
3. Enriching educational programs, which will be given to the children after school hours, such as music, art, sports, and working with computers.
4. A center for adult education and occupational training that can open up job alternatives for adults.
5. Coordination between specific services, such as rehabilitation centers for substance abuse, probation officers, and the social services department. Such coordination reduces competition between services to the benefit of the client.
6. Where policy allows it, an FED center is recommended (see Figure 12.2).

FIGURE 12.2. The FED Center

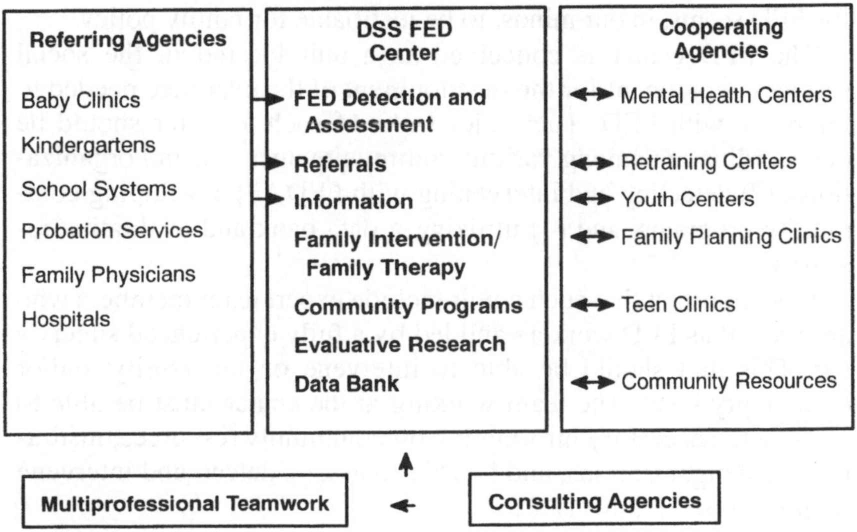

Before discussing an FED center, let us look at the concept of family policy and how it relates to FED.

Kamerman and Kahn (1978) define family policy as "everything that government does to or for the family," whether explicit or implicit, intended or unintended. They include in their definition of family policy those governmental actions and policies not specifically addressed to the family, but still affecting it (Kamerman and Kahn, 1978). McDonald (1979) points out that although most public policy is directed toward individuals, it affects not only individuals but the families to which they belong as well.

Family policy can go in several possible directions. One recommended direction is to focus on certain types of families. Bane (1980) suggests families with children; Kahn and Kamerman (1978) point to the aged, women, and children. In addition to target populations, some emphasize important areas such as family health, emotional state, financial condition, and culture. Aldous and Dumon (1990) recommend that family policy should stress economic dimensions related to families with children. Still others highlight families with a large number of children. Our experience in the FED project leads us to believe that family policy is a valuable tool, a systematic perspective within social policy that can be used to focus objectives on quality of life. Thus, building a specific program through a project for FED seems, in our minds, to be justifiable for family policy.

The FED center is conceived as a unit located in the social services department for the development of the expertise needed to intervene with FED. The major tasks of such a center should be (1) coordinating among various community agencies and organizations, (2) detecting and intervening with FED, (3) developing community programs, and (4) utilizing a data bank and evaluative research.

It is important that such a unit include expert team members who are trained as FED workers and led by a fully experienced supervisor. This unit should be able to intervene on the family and/or community level. The team working at the center must be able to provide the necessary information on community resources, institutions and organizations, and be able to assess, detect, and intervene with FED (see Figure 12.2).

Referring agencies comprise all relevant agencies in a given community, some of which may be later involved as part of the multiprofessional teamwork. Cooperating agencies operate independently in a given community and may serve either as referral agencies or in the capacity of consultants to the FED center in treating FED. The FED center can also develop self-help programs, possibly headed by a member of an FED family. This will empower FED family members and reveal their hidden strengths in problem solving and in taking on and managing responsibility. The case of Mrs. S. is a good example.

It is important to keep in mind that the cost of intervention and follow-up with FED is far more expensive than prevention. The FED center can provide experts in early detection of families at risk and in preventive programs. Let us take a look at a possible scenario of an FED left untreated. It is most likely that life in such a family would deteriorate and that the family would eventually break up. Subsequent costs for social services, the court system, foster care and institutions, and various other professionals involved in the decision-making process would be enormous. Early detection and prevention, however, may save a major part of the cost of intervention.

When suggesting a permanent FED center, one may wonder about the effectiveness of a single project with FED. We have found that such a unique project contributes in various ways. For one, it makes some noise within the system, highlighting the very concept of FED. There has been some enthusiasm for this new approach, but it will not last forever, especially when working with such a complex population. Therefore, it is good to keep in mind the benefits as well as the limitations of a permanent FED center.

Finally, we would like to add a personal comment. We were very enthusiastic about getting involved with FED. Despite our limited financial resources, we had infinite curiosity, motivation, and hope, and we succeeded in transferring our enthusiasm to those who took part in this project, namely, the therapeutic team and the client families. Such enthusiasm sustained us in our search for ways to join with the families in creating hope. It turned out that hope, as a resource, was most effective in bringing about the changes that the families achieved through intervention.

Bibliography

Ackerly, S. (1947). The clinical team. *American Journal of Orthopsychiatry* 17:191-195.

Aldous, I. and Dumon, W. (1990). Family policy in the 1980s: Controversy and consensus. *Journal of Marriage and the Family* 52:1136-1151.

Alexander, J.F. (1973). Defensive and supportive communication in normal and deviant families. *Journal of Consulting and Clinical Psychology* 4:223-231.

Alexander, J.F. and Parsons, B.V. (1973). Short-term behavioral intervention with delinquent families: Impact on family process and recidivism. *Journal of Abnormal Psychology* 81(3):219-225.

Amundson, J., Stewart, K., and Valentine, L. (1993). Temptations of power and certainty. *Journal of Marital and Family Therapy* 32:111-123.

Anderson, C.M. (1988). The selection of measures in family therapy research. In L.C. Wynne (Ed.), *The State of the art in family therapy research—Controversies and recommendations* (pp. 81-87). Rochester, NY: Family Process Press.

Anderson, G.L. (1992). Dissociation, distress and family function. *Dissociation: Progress in the Dissociative Disorders* 5(4):210-215.

Andrews, J.A., Lewinsohn, P.M., Hops, H., and Roberts, R.E. (1993). Psychometric properties of scales for the measurement of psychosocial variables associated with depression in adolescence. *Psychological Reports* 73(3, part 1): 1019-1046.

Auerwald, E.H. (1972). Families, change and the ecological perspective. In A. Ferber, M. Mendelson, and A. Napier (Eds.), *The book of family therapy* (pp. 684-705). Boston: Houghton Mifflin.

Aponte, H. (1974a). Organizing treatment around the family's problems and their structural bases. *Psychiatric Quarterly* 48:209-222.

Aponte, H. (1974b). Psychotherapy for the poor: An ecostructural approach to treatment. *Delaware Medical Journal* 46:134-144.

Aponte, H. (1976a). Underorganization in the poor family. In P. Guerin Jr. (Ed.), *Family therapy theory and practice* (pp. 432-448). New York: Gardner Press.

Aponte, H. (1976b). The family school interview: An eco-structural approach. *Family Process* 15(3):303-311.

Aponte, H. (1979a). Family therapy and the community. In M.S. Gibbs, J.R. Lachemeyer, and G. Sigal (Eds.), *Community psychology—The oretical and empirical approaches* (pp. 311-333). New York: Gardner Press.

Aponte, H. (1979b). Diagnosis in family therapy. In C.B. Germain (Ed.), *Social work practice: People and environments* (pp. 107-149). New York: Columbia University Press.

Aponte, H. (1982). The cornerstone of therapy: The person of the therapist. *Family Therapy Networker* 6:19-21.

Aponte, H. (1985a). The negotiation of values in therapy. *Family Process* 24:323-338.

Aponte, H. (1985b). Adolescent acting out when a parent has cancer: Discussion. *International Journal of Family Therapy* 7(3):176-177.

Aponte, H. (1986). If I don't get simple, I cry. *Family Process* 25(4):531-548.

Aponte, H. (1989). Please join me in a short walk through the South Bronx. *AFTA Newsletter* 37:36-40.

Aponte, H. (1990). Too many bosses: An ecostructural intervention with a family and its community. *Journal of Strategic and Systemic Therapies* 9(3):49-63.

Aponte, H. (1991). Training on the person of the therapist for work with the poor and minorities. *Journal of Independent Social Work* 5(3/4):23-39.

Aponte, H. (1994). *Bread and spirit: Therapy with the new poor, diversity of race, culture and values.* New York: W. W. Norton and Company.

Aponte, R. (1993). Hispanic families in poverty: Diversity, context and interpretation. *Families in Society* 74:527-537.

Aram, E. (nd). *Dror—Breaking the chain of distress.* A paper presented in a special program organized by the JDC for children at risk and their parents. Unpublished manuscript.

Argles, P. and MacKenzie, M. (1970). Crisis intervention with a multiproblem family: A case study. *Journal of Child Psychology and Psychiatry and Applied Disciplines* 11:187-195.

Armstrong, R. and Reigeluth, C.M. (1991). The TIP theory: Prescriptions for designing instructions for teams. *Performance Improvement Quarterly* 4(3):13-40.

Arndt, H.C.M. (1955). Principles of supervision in public assistance agencies. *Social Casework* 36:307-313.

Aronson, O. (1966). Treatment expectations of patients in two social classes. *Social Work* 11:35-41.

Atkinson, B.J. (1993). Hierarchy: The imbalance of risk. *Family Process* 32:167-170.

Baker, D. and Salas, E. (1992). Principles for measuring teamwork skills. Special issue: Measurement in human factors. *Human Factors* 34(4):469-475.

Bandler, R. and Grinder, J. (1979). *Frogs into process: Neurolinguistic programming.* Moab, UT: Real People Press.

Bandura, A. (1977). Self-efficacy: Towards a unifying theory of behavioral change. *Psychological Review* 23:191-215.

Bane, M.J. (1980). Towards a description and evaluation of United States family policy. In J. Aldous and W. Dumon (Eds.), *The politics and programs of family policy: United States and European perspectives* (pp. 155-191). Notre Dame, IN: University of Notre Dame Press.

Bergin, A.E. and Lambert, M.J. (1978). The evaluation of therapeutic outcomes. In S.L. Garfield and A.E. Bergin (Eds.), *Handbook of psychotherapy and behavior change: An empirical analysis* (pp. 139-189). New York: John Wiley and Sons.

Bernstein, B. (1960). Language and social class. *British Journal of Sociology* 11:271-276.

Bernstein, B. (1961). Social class and linguistic development: A theory of social learning. In A.H. Halsey, J. Floud, and C.A. Anderson (Eds.), *Education economy and society* (pp. 288-314). New York: The Free Press of Glencoe.

Bernstein, B. (1962). Social class, linguistic codes and grammatical elements. *Language Speech* 5:221-240.

Bernstein, B. (1964). Social class, speech systems and psychotherapy. *British Journal of Sociology* 15:54-64.

Bernstein, V.J., Jeremy, R.J., and Marcus, H. (1986). Mother-infant interactions in multiproblem families: Finding those at risk. *Journal of American Academy of Child Psychiatry* 25:631-640.

Berry, J., Hurley, J., Everett, L., and Worthington, R. (1990). Empirical validity of the Kvebaek family sculpture technique. *The American Journal of Family Therapy* 18(1):19-31.

Billingsley, A. (1969). Family functioning in the low-income black community. *Social Casework* 50:563-572.

Birt, C.J. (1956). Family Centered Project of St. Paul. *Social Work* 1:41-47.

Booth, C. (1903). *Life and labour of the people in London.* London: Macmillan and Company.

Borden, W. (1992). Narrative perspectives in psychosocial intervention following adverse life events. *Social Work* 37(2):135-141.

Boscolo, L., Cecchin, G., Hoffman, L., and Penn, P. (1987). *Milan systemic therapy.* New York: Basic Books.

Bowen, M. (1976). Theory in the practice of psychotherapy. In P. Guerin (Ed.), *Family therapy: Theory and practice* (pp. 42-90). New York: Gardner Press.

Boyd-Franklin, N. (1989). *Black families in therapy: A multisystems approach.* New York: Guilford Press.

Brill, N.I. (1976). *Teamwork: Working together in the human services.* New York: J.B. Lippincott Company.

Brodley, B.T. (1989). Client-centered and experiential: Two different therapies. In G. Lietaer, J. Rombants, and R. Van-Balen (Eds.), *Client-centered and experiential psychotherapy in the nineties* (pp. 97-107). Leuven, Belgium: Leuven University Press.

Bronfenbrenner, U. (1968). *Motivational and social components in compensatory education programs, suggested principles, practice and research designs.* Washington, DC: Office of Education.

Brossman, M. (1990). Home-based family therapy not same as office practice. Part 1. In R. Cassano (Ed.), *Social work with multi family groups.* Binghamton, NY: The Haworth Press, Inc.

Bruno, F.J. (1948). *Trends in Social Work, 1874-1956.* New York: Columbia University Press.

Bryce, M. and Lloyd, J.C. (Eds.) (1981). *Treating families in-home: An alternative to placement.* Springfield, IL: Charles C Thomas.

Buell, B. and associates (1952). *Community planning for human services*. New York: Columbia University Press.

Bulehorn, L. (1978). A plan for identifying priorities in treating multi-problem families. *Child Welfare* 57:365-372.

Burnham, D.K. (1993). Visual recognition of mother by young infants: Facilitation by speech. *Perception* 22(10):1133-1153.

Burnham, D.K. and Harris, M.B. (1992). Effects of real gender and labeled genders on adults' perceptions of infants. *Journal of Genetic Psychology* 153(2):165-183.

Burt, M.R. (1976a). The comprehensive emergency system: Expanding services to children and families. *Children Today* 5(2):2-5.

Burt, M.R. (1976b). Final results of Nashville Comprehensive Emergency Services Project. *Child Welfare* 55:661-664.

Butcher, J.N. and Ross, M.P. (1978). Research on brief and crisis oriented psychotherapies. In S.L. Garfield and A.E. Bergin (Eds.), *Handbook of psychotherapy and behavior change: An empirical analysis* (pp. 725-767). New York: John Wiley and Sons.

Cade, B. (1975). Therapy with the low socio-economic families. *Social Work Today* 6:142-145.

Chilman, C.S. (1966). Social work practice with very poor families: Some implications and suggestions from research. *Welfare in Review* 4:13-22.

Chilman, C.S. (1968). Poor families and their patterns of child care: Some implications for service programs. In L. Dittman (Ed.), *Early child care: The new perspectives* (pp. 217-236). New York: Atherton Press.

Chilman, C.S. (1973). Some psychological aspects of fertility, family planning and population policy in the United States. In J. Fawcett (Ed.), *Psychological perspectives on population* (pp. 163-181). New York: Basic Books.

Clark, K.B. (1965). *Dark ghetto: Dilemmas of social power.* New York: Harper & Row.

Compler, J.V. (1983). Home services to families to prevent child placement. *Social Work* 28:360-364.

Compton, B.R. (1962). *The Family Centered Project.* Paper presented at the annual meeting of the Children's Aid Society of Winnipeg, Manitoba, Canada, April 25, 1962.

Compton, B.R. (1979). *The Family Centered Project Revisited.* Minneapolis, MN: School of Social Work, University of Minnesota, May.

Conger, K.J. and Conger, R.D. (1994). Differential parenting and change in sibling differences in delinquency. *Journal of Family Psychology* 8(3):287-302.

Craig, B. and Hurry, D. (1981). Rural multiproblem families. *Journal of Family Therapy* 3:91-99.

Cromwell, R., Fournier, D., and Kvebaek, D. (1980). *The Kvebaek family sculpture technique: A diagnostic and research tool in family therapy.* Jonesboro, TN: Pilgrimage, USA.

Dax, E.C. and Hagger, R. (1977). Multiproblem families and their psychiatric significance. *Australian and New Zealand Journal of Psychiatry* 11:227-232.

de Shazer, S. (1985). *Keys to solution in brief therapy.* New York: Norton.

Deutch, M. (1963). The disadvantaged child and the learning process. In A.H. Passow (Ed.), *Education in depressed areas* (pp. 163-179). New York: Bureau of Publications, Teachers College, Columbia University.

Deutch, M. (1965). The role of social class in language development and cognition. *American Journal of Orthopsychiatry* 35:78-88.

Dewey, I. (1933). Analysis of reflective thinking. In: *How do we think?* New York: D.C. Health and Company.

Dodge, K.A., Pettit, G., and Bates, J.E. (1994). Socialization mediators of the relation between socioeconomic status and child conduct problems. *Child Development* 65(2):649-665.

Dohrenwend, B.S. and Dohrenwend, B.P. (1981). Hypotheses about stress process linking social class to various types of psychopathology. *American Journal of Community Psychology* 9:146-159.

Ducanis, A.J. and Golin, A.K. (1979). *The interdisciplinary health care team. A handbook.* London: Aspen System Corporation.

Dumas, J.E. and Wekerle, C. (1995). Maternal reports of child behavior problems and personal distress as predictors of dysfunctional parenting. *Development and Psychopathology* 7(3):465-479.

Duncan, D.F. (1996). Growing up under the gun: Children and adolescents coping with violent neighborhoods. *Journal of Primary Prevention* 16(4):343-356.

Duncan, G.J., Brooks-Gunn, J., and Klebanov, P.K. (1994). Economic deprivation and early childhood development. *Child Development* 65(2):296-318.

Ecklad, G. and Vandvik, H. (1992). A computerized scoring procedure for the Kvebaek family sculpture technique applied to families of children with rheumatic diseases. *Family Process* 31:85-98.

Elkaim, M. (1997). *If you love me, don't love me.* Northdale, NJ: Jason Aronson.

Epstein, E.B., Baldwin, L.M., and Bishop, D.S. (1983). The McMaster family assessment device. *Journal of Marital and Family Therapy* 9(2):171-180.

Epstein, N., Bishop, D.S., and Baldwin, L.M. (1982). McMaster model of family functioning: A view of the normal family. In F. Walsh (Ed.), *Normal family processes* (pp. 115-141). New York: Guilford Press.

Erera, I.P. (1983). *Burnout and role stress among social work supervisors.* Doctoral dissertation, Cornell University.

Eron, J.B. and Lund T.W. (1993). How problems evolve and dissolve: Integrating narrative and strategic concepts. *Family Process* 32(3):291-309.

Eysenck, H.J. (1952). The effects of psychotherapy: An evaluation. *Journal of Consulting Psychology* 16:319-324.

Famularo, R., Kinscherff, R., and Fenton, T. (1992). Psychiatric diagnoses of maltreated children: Preliminary findings. *Journal of the American Academy of Child and Adolescent Psychiatry* 31(5):863-867.

Farrington, D.P. (1990). Implications of criminal career research for the prevention of offending. *Journal of Adolescence* 13(2):93-113.

Feldman, Y. (1977). The supervisory process: An experience in teaching and learning. *Studies in Social Work* 47:154-161.

Fischer, J. (1978). *Effective casework practice: An eclectic approach.* New York: McGraw-Hill.
Frairberg, S. (1978). Psychoanalysis and social work: A reexamination of the issues. *Social Work* 48(2):87-106.
Frankenstein, K. (1969). *Youth on the margin of society.* Tel Aviv, Israel: Achiasaf.
Freud, S. (1950). *Collected Papers,* Volume I. London: Hogarth Press and the Institute of Psychoanalysis.
Friesen, D. and Sarros, J. (1981). Sources of burnout among educators. *Journal of Organizational Behavior* 10:179-188.
Galbraith, J.K. (1958). *The affluent society.* London: Hamish Hamilton.
Gans, H.G. (1963). Social and physical planning for the elimination of urban poverty. *Washington University Law Quarterly* 2:18.
Garcia-Preto, N. (1982). Puerto Rican families. In M. McGoldrik, J.K. Pearce, and J. Giordano (Eds.), *Ethnicity and family therapy* (pp. 183-199). New York: Guilford Press.
Gatti, F. and Colman, C. (1976). Community network therapy: An approach to aiding families with troubled children. *American Journal of Orthopsychiatry* 46:608-617.
Gawin, F.H. and Ellinwood, E. (1988). Cocaine and other stimulants: Actions, abuse and treatment. *New England Journal of Medicine* 318(18):1173-1182.
Geismar, L.L. (1971a). Implications of Family Life Improvement Project, *Social Casework* 52:455-465.
Geismar, L.L. (1971b). *Family and community functioning: A manual of measurement for social work practice and policy.* Metuchen, NJ: The Scarecrow Press.
Geismar, L. (1973). *555 families: A social psychology study of young families in transition.* New Brunswick, NJ: Transaction Books (Dutton).
Geismar, L.L. and Krisberg, J. (1967). *The forgotten neighborhood: Site of an early skirmish in the war on poverty.* Metuchen, NJ: The Scarecrow Press.
Geismar, L.L. and La Sorte, M.A. (1964). *Understanding the multi-problem family: A conceptual analysis and exploration in early identification.* New York: Association Press.
Gilad-Smolinsky, D. (1996). Method of therapy treatment intervention with families suffering from severe and deep distress. MA thesis submitted to the University of Haifa.
Goldstein, H. (1973). Providing services to children in their own homes. *Children Today* 2:2-7.
Gorman, S.D. (1996). Prospects and possibilities: Next steps in sound understanding of youth violence. *Journal of Family Psychology* 10(2):153-157.
Grotevant, H.D. and Carlson, C.I. (1989). *Family assessment: A guide to methods and measures.* New York: Guilford Press.
Haley, J. (1976). *Problem-solving therapy.* San Francisco: Jossey-Bass.
Hanson, M.S. and Carta, J.J. (1996). Addressing the challenges of families with multiple risks. *Exceptional Children* 62(3):201-212.
Hardy-Fanta, C. and MacMahon-Herrera E. (1981). Adapting family therapy to the Hispanic family. *Social Casework* 62:138-148.

Harrington, M. (1962). *The other America: Poverty in the United States.* New York: Macmillan.

Harvey, D.M. and Bray, J.H. (1991). Evaluation of an intergenerational theory of personal development: Family process determinants of psychological and health distress. *Journal of Family Psychology* 4(3):298-325.

Henggeler, S.W., Borduin C.M., Melton, G., and Mann, B.L. (1991). Effects of multisystemic therapy on drug use and abuse in serious juvenile offenders: A progress report from two outcome studies. *Family Dynamics of Addiction Quarterly* 1(3):40-51.

Heying, K.R. (1985). Family-based, in-home services for the severely emotionally disturbed child. *Child Welfare* 64:519-527.

Holland, A.J. (1991). Challenging and offending behavior by adults with developmental disorders. *Australia and New Zealand Journal of Developmental Disabilities* 17(2):119-126.

Jones, N.A., Neuman, R., and Shyne, A.W. (1976). *A second chance for families: Evaluation of program to reduce foster care.* New York: Child Welfare League of America.

Kadushin, A. (1985). *Supervision in social work.* New York: Columbia University Press.

Kamerman, S.B. and Kahn, A.J. (Eds.) (1978). *Family policy: Government and families in fourteen countries.* New York: Columbia University Press.

Kaplan, L.W. (1984). The multi-problem family phenomenon: An interactional perspective. A PhD dissertation submitted to the graduate school of the University of Massachusetts.

Kaplan, L.W. (1986). *Working with multi-problem families.* Lexington, MA: Lexington Books.

Kaslow, F.W. (1986). *Supervision and training.* Binghamton, NY: The Haworth Press, Inc.

Kaslow, F.W. (1995). Nobody's children or everybody's children. In William J. O'Neill Jr. (Ed.), *Family: The first imperative.* Ohio: The William and Dorothy K. O'Neill Foundation.

Kim-Berg, I. (1991). *Family preservation: A brief therapy workbook.* London: B.T. Press.

Ki-Tov, Y. and Ben-David, A. (1993). The cultural component in marital therapy with immigrants from Ethiopia. *Society and Welfare* 13(3):265-278.

Kuperminc, G.P. and Repucci, N.D. (1996). Contributions of new research on juvenile delinquency to the prevention and treatment of antisocial behavior. *Journal of Family Psychology* 19(2):130-136.

Leinwand, G. (1968). *Poverty and the poor.* New York: Washington Square Press.

Levine, R.A. (1964). Treatment in the home. *Social Work* 9(1):19-28.

Lewis, O. (1959). *Five families.* New York: Basic Books.

Lewis, O. (1961). *The children of Sanchez.* New York: Random House.

Lewis, O. (1966). The culture of poverty. *Scientific American* 215(4):19-25.

Long, J.V. and Vaillant, G.E. (1984). Natural history of male psychological health. XI: Escape from the underclass. *American Journal of Psychiatry* 141(3):341-346.

Lorion, R.P. (1973). Socioeconomic status and traditional treatment approaches reconsidered. *Psychological Bulletin* 79:263-240.

Lorion, R.P. (1974). Patient and therapist variables in the treatment of low income patients. *Psychological Bulletin* 81:344-354.

Lorion, R.P. (1978). Research on psychotherapy and behavior change with the disadvantaged: Past, present and future directions. In S.L. Garfield and A.E. Bergen (Eds.), *Handbook of psychotherapy and behavior change: An empirical analysis* (pp. 903-938). New York: John Wiley and Sons.

Lowe, J.L. and Herranen, M. (1981). Understanding teamwork: Another look at the concepts. *Social Work in Health Care* 7(2):1-11.

Madanes, C. (1981). *Strategic family therapy.* San Franciso: Jossey-Bass.

Madanes, C. (1986). *Behind the one-way mirror.* San Francisco: Jossey-Bass.

Magura, S. (1981). Are services to prevent foster care effective? *Children and Youth Services Review* 3:193-212.

Mallucio, A.N. and Marlow, W.P. (1974). The case for the contract. *Social Work* 19:28-36.

Marans, A.E. and Lourie, R. (1967). Hypotheses regarding the effects of child rearing patterns on the disadvantaged child. In J. Hellmuth (Ed.), *The Disadvantaged Child,* Volume 1. Seattle, WA: Special Child Publications.

Marshall, M., Person-Shoot, M., and Winnicott, E. (Eds.) (1979). *Teamwork for and against: An appraisal of multi-disciplinary practice.* Birmingham, England: BASW Publications.

Maslach, C. and Pines, A. (1977). Burnout, the loss of human caring. In A. Pines and C. Maslach (Eds.), *Experiencing social psychology.* New York: Random House.

Maybanks, S. and Bryce, M. (Eds.) (1979). *Home-based services for children and families: Policy, practice and research.* Springfield, IL: Charles C Thomas.

Mazer, M. (1972). Characteristic of multi-problem households: A study in psychosocial epidemiology. *American Journal of Orthopsychiatry* 42:792-802.

McCord, J. (1996). Family as crucible for violence. *Journal of Family Psychology* 10(2):147-152.

McDaniel, S. and Campbell, T. (1986). Physicians and family therapists: The risk of collaboration. *Family Systems Medicine* 4(1):4-8.

McDonald, G.W. (1979). Typology for family policy research. *Social Work* 24(6): 553-559.

McGowan, B.G. and Meesan, W. (1983). *Child welfare: Current dilemmas, future directions.* Itasca, IL: F. E. Peacock.

McLoyd, V.C. (1989). Socialization and development in a changing economy: The effects of paternal job and income loss on children. *American Psychologist* 44(2):293-302.

McLoyd, V.C. (1990). Maternal behavior, social support and economic conditions as predictors of distress in children. *New Directions for Child Development* 46:49-69.

McMahan, E.M., Hoffman, K., and McGee, G.W. (1994). Physican-nurse relationships in clinical settings: A review and critique of the literature 1966-1992. *Medical Care Review* 51(1):83-112.

McNamee, S. and Gergen, K.J. (1992). *Therapy as social construction.* Thousand Oaks, CA: Sage.

Meyer, A.A. (1995). Minimization of substance use: What can be paid at this part. In T.P. Guillotta, G.R. Adams, and A.J. Hontemayer (Eds.), *Substance misuse in adolescence* (pp. 201-232). Thousand Oaks, CA: Sage.

Meyer, C.H. (1963). Individualizing the multiproblem family. *Social Casework* 44:267-272.

Miller, I.W., Epstein, N.B., Bishop, D.S., and Keitner, G.I. (1985). The McMaster family assessment device: Reliability and validity. *Journal of Marital and Family Therapy* 11(1):345-356.

Miller, W.B. (1962). *Cultural factors of an urban lower class community.* Silver Spring, MD: National Institute of Mental Health, Community Services Branch.

Minuchin, S. (1970). The plight of the poverty-stricken family in the United States. *Child Welfare* 49:124-130.

Minuchin, S. (1974). *Families and family therapy.* Cambridge, MA: Harvard University Press.

Minuchin, S. and Fishman, G.H. (1981). *Family therapy techniques.* Cambridge, MA: Harvard University Press.

Minuchin, S. and Montalvo, B. (1968). Techniques for working with disorganized low socioeconomic families. *American Journal of Orthopsychiatry* 37: 880-887.

Minuchin, S., Montalvo, B., Guerney, B.G., Rosman, B.L., and Shumer, F. (1967). *Families of the slums: An exploration of their structure and treatment.* New York: Basic Books.

Mostwin, D. (1980). *Social dimension of family treatment.* Washington, DC: National Association for Social Workers.

Munroe-Blum, H., Boyle, M.H., and Offord, D.R. (1988). Single-parent families: Child psychiatric disorder and school performance. *Journal of the American Academy of Child and Adolescent Psychiatry* 27:214-219.

Munson, C.E. (1983). *An introduction to clinical social work supervision.* Binghamton, NY: The Haworth Press, Inc.

Needleman, H.L., Schell, A., Bellinger, D., and Leviton, A. (1990). The long-term effect of exposure to low doses of lead in childhood: An eleven-year follow-up report. *New England Journal of Medicine* 322(2):83-88.

O'Hanlon, W.H. (1991). Foreword. In J.E. Gale (Ed.), *Conversation analysis of therapeutic discourse: Pursuit of a therapeutic agenda* (pp. ix-x). Norwood, NJ: Ablex.

O'Hanlon, W.H. and Weiner-Davis, M. (1989). *In search of solutions: A new direction in psychotherapy.* New York: W. W. Norton.

Olson, D.H., Portner, J., and Lavee, Y. (1985). *Faces III.* St. Paul, MN: Family Social Science, University of Minnesota.

Olson, D.H., Sprenkle, D.H., and Russell, C.S. (1979). Circumplex model of marital and family systems: Cohesion and adaptability dimensions, family types and clinical applications. *Family Process* 18:3-28.

Papp, P. (1983). *The process of change*. New York: Guilford.

Parry, A. and Doan, R.E. (1994). *Story revisions: Narrative therapy in the post-modern world.* New York: Guilford.

Parsons, B.V. and Alexander, J.F. (1973). Short-term family intervention: A therapy outcome study. *Journal of Consulting and Clinical Psychology* 41(2):195-201.

Pasamanick, B. (Ed.) (1959). *Epidemiology of mental disorders.* Washington, DC: The American Association for the Advancement of Science.

Patterson, G.R. (1972). *A social learning approach: Coercive family process.* Eugene, OR: Castalia.

Patterson, G.R. and Bank, L. (1986). Bootstrapping your way in the nomological thicket. *Behavioral Assessment* 8(1):49-73.

Patterson, G.R. and Bank, L.C. (1989). Some amplifying mechanisms for pathological processes in families. In M.R. Gunnar and E. Thelen (Eds.), *Systems and development: The Minnesota symposia on child psychology,* Volume 22 (pp. 167-209). Hillsdale, NJ: Lawrence Erlbaum Associates, Inc.

Patterson, G.R., Crosby, L., and Vuchinich, S. (1992). Predicting risk for early police arrest. *Journal of Quantitative Criminology* 8(4):335-355.

Pavenstedt, E. (1965). A comparison of the child-rearing environment of upper-lower and very low-lower class families. *American Journal of Orthopsychiatry* 35:89-98.

Pavenstedt, E. (Ed.) (1967). *The drifters: Children of disorganized lower-class families.* Boston: Little Brown.

Pearl, A. and Riessman, F. (1965). *New careers for the poor: The nonprofessional in human services.* New York: The Free Press.

Pettigrew, T.F. (1964). *A profile of the Negro American.* Toronto, Canada: Princeton, Nostrand.

Pinkston, E., Levitt, J.L., Green, G.R., Linsk, N.L., and Rzepnicki, T.L. (1982). *Effective social work practice: Advanced techniques for behavioral intervention with individuals, families and institutional staff.* San Francisco: Jossey-Bass.

Polansky, N.A. (1965). The concept of verbal accessibility. *Smith College Studies in Social Work* 36(1):1-48.

Polansky, N.A. (1971). *Egopsychology and communication.* Chicago: Aldine.

Polansky, N.A. (1986). There is nothing so practical as a good theory. *Child Welfare* LXV(1): 1-15.

Polansky, N.A., Borgman, R.D., and DeSaix, C. (1972). *Roots of futility.* San Francisco: Jossey-Bass.

Polansky, N.A., Borgman, R.D., DeSaix, C., and Smith, B.J. (1970). Two models of maternal immaturity and their consequences. *Child Welfare* 49:312-323.

Polansky, N.A., Chalmers, M.A., Buttewieser, E., and Williams, D.P. (1981). *Damaged parents: An anatomy of child neglect.* Chicago and London: The University of Chicago Press.

Polansky, N.A., DeSaix, C., and Sharlin, S.A. (1972). *Child neglect: Understanding and teaching the parent.* New York: Child Welfare League of America.

Rabin, C. (1989). Gender issues in the treatment of welfare couples: A feminist approach to marital therapy of the poor. *Contemporary Family Therapy: An International Journal* 11:169-178.

Rabin, C., Rosenbaum, H., and Sens, M. (1982). Home-based marital therapy for multi-problem families. *Journal of Marital and Family Therapy* 8:451-461.

Reid, W. (1987). Research in social work. In K.R. Greenhall (Ed.), *Encyclopedia of social work,* Volume 2 (pp. 474-487). Silver Spring, MD: National Association of Social Workers.

Reid, W. and Smith, A. (1981). *Research in social work.* New York: Columbia University Press.

Riessman, F. (1967). Strategies and suggestions for training nonprofessionals. *Community Mental Health* 3:103-110.

Riessman, F., Cohen, J., and Pearl, H. (Eds.) (1964). *Mental health of the poor.* New York: Free Press.

Rivara, F.P. and Mueller, B.A. (1987). The epidemiology and causes of childhood injuries. *Journal of Social Issues* 43(2):13-31.

Ronnau, J.P. and Marlow, C.R. (1993). Family preservation, poverty and the value of diversity. *Families in Society* 74(9):538-544.

Rosenfeld, J.M. (1989). *Emergence from extreme poverty.* Paris: Science et Service, Fourth World Publications.

Rosenfeld, J.M., Schor, D.A., and Sykes, I.J. (1995). *Out from under.* Jerusalem: JDC—Brookdale Institute of Gerontology and Human Development.

Rosenthal, A.P., Mosteller, S., Wells, J.L., and Rolland, R.S. (1974). Family therapy with multi-problem, multi-children families in a court clinic setting, *Journal of the American Academy of Child Psychiatry* 13:126-142.

Rutter, M. (1981). Social emotional consequences of day care for preschool children. *American Journal of Orthopsychiatry* 51(1):4-28.

Ryan, D.P. (1996). A history of teamwork in mental health and its implications for teamwork training and education in gerontology. *Educational Gerontology* 22(5):411-431.

Saleebey, D. (Ed.) (1992). *The strength perspective in social work practice.* New York: Longman.

Sampson, R.L. and Laub, J.H. (1994). Urban poverty and the family context of delinquency: A new look at structure and process in a classic study. *Child Development* 65(2):523-540.

Satir, V. (1972). *Conjoint family therapy.* Palo Alto, CA: Science and Behavior Books.

Satir, V.M. and Baldwin, M. (1983). *Satir step by step: A guide to creating change in families.* Palto Alto, CA: Science and Behavior Books.

Schiff, M. and Kalter, N. (1980). The multi-problem family parents in children's outpatient psychiatric clinic. *Advances in Family Psychiatry* 20:533-543.

Schlesinger, B. (1963). *The multi-problem family: A review and annotated bibliography.* Toronto, Canada: University of Toronto Press.

Schlesinger, B. (1970). The multi-problem family in Canada: A glance backward. In Schlesinger, B. (Ed.), *The multi-problem family: A review and annotated bibliography* (pp. 73-87). Toronto, Canada: University of Toronto Press.

Schlosberg, S. and Kagan, R. (1988). Practice strategies for engaging chronic multiproblem families. *Social Casework* 69:3-9.

Scott, J.A. (1956). *Appendix on problem families in London.* London: London County Council, Public Health Department.

Seabury, B.A. (1976). The contract: Uses, abuses and limitations. *Social Work* 21:16-21.

Selvini-Pallazoli, M., Boscolo, L., Cecchin, G., and Prata, G. (1978). *Paradox and counter-paradox.* New York: Jason Aronson.

Sexton, P.C. (1965). *Spanish Harlem: Anatomy of poverty.* New York: Harper & Row.

Shamai, M. (1987). Structured contract vs. general agreement. PhD dissertation submitted to the School of Social Service Administration at the University of Chicago.

Shamai, M. and Sharlin, S.A. (1996). Who writes the "therapeutic story" of families in extreme distress: Overcoming the coalition of despair. *Journal of Family Social Work* 1:65-82.

Shapiro, A.K. and Morris, L.A. (1978). Placebo effects in medical and psychological therapies. In S.L. Garfield and A.R. Bergin (Eds.), *Handbook of psychotherapy and behavior change: An empirical analysis* (pp. 369-410). New York: John Wiley and Sons.

Sharlin, S.A. and Chaiklin, H. (1998). The social work education field experience. *The Clinical Supervisor* 17(1):1-16.

Sharlin, S.A. and Elshansky, I. (1997). Parental attitudes of Soviets in Israel to the immigration process and their impact on parental stress and tension. In S. Dreman (Ed.), *The family on the threshold of the 21st century: Trends and implications.* Mahwah, NJ: Lawrence Erlbaum.

Sharlin, S.A., Katz, R., and Lavee, Y. (1992). Families in Israel in the year 2000. *Society and Welfare* 12(2):167-187.

Sharlin, S.A. and Shamai, M. (1990). *Families in extreme distress (FED)—Identification and intervention.* Haifa, Israel: The Center for Research and Study of the Family, University of Haifa.

Sharlin, S.A. and Shamai, M. (1995). Intervention with families in extreme distress (FED). *Marriage and Family Review* 21:92-122.

Sharlin, S.A., Shamai, M., and Gilad-Smolinsky, D. (1994). The therapeutic challenge of working with families in extreme distress (FED)—A case study. *Journal of Family Psychotherapy* 5(1):21-39.

Sharlin, S.A., Shamai, M., and Gilad-Smolinsky, D. (1995). Using a threat of divorce for maintaining family homeostasis within families in extreme distress (FED). *Contemporary Family Therapy* 17(2):195-207.

Sharlin, S.A. and Shenhar-Alroy, A. (1987). *On adolescent suicide and poetry: An approach for early detection.* King George, VA: American Foster Care Resources.

Shaw, D.S., Vondra, J.I., Hommerding, K.D., and Keenan, K. (1994). Chronic family adversity and early child behaviour problems: A longitudinal study of low income families. *Journal of Child Psychology and Psychiatry and Allied Disciplines* 35:1109-1122.

Shlein, J.M., Mosak, M.H., and Dreikurs, R. (1962). Effects on time-limits: A comparison of two psychotherapies. *Journal of Counseling Psychology* 9:31-34.

Skurray, G. and Ham, R. (1990). Family poverty and child abuse. *Australian Journal of Marriage and the Family* 11:94-99.

Spencer, J. (1963a). *Stress and release in an urban estate.* London: Tavistock Publications.

Spencer, J. (1963b). The multi-problem family. In B. Schlesinger (Ed.), *The multi-problem family: A review and annotated bibliography* (pp. 3-54). Toronto, Canada: University of Toronto Press.

Sprenkle, D.H. and Piercy, F.P. (1992). A family therapy informed view of the current state of the family in the United States. *Family Relation* 41(4):404-408.

Stuart, R.B., (1980). *Helping couples change: A social learning approach to marital therapy.* Champaign, IL: Research Press.

Tarnowski, K.J. and Rohrbeck, C.A. (1993). Disadvantaged children and families. *Advances in Clinical Child Psychology* 15:41-79.

Tavantzis, T.N., Tavantzis, M., Brown, L.G., and Rohrbough, M. (1985). Home-based family therapy for delinquents at risk of placement. In M.P. Mirkin and S. Koman (Eds.), *Handbook of adolescents and family therapy* (pp. 69-88). New York: Gardner.

Tolan, P.H. and Loeber, R. (1993). Antisocial behavior. In P.H. Tolan and B.J. Cohler (Eds.), *Handbook of clinical research and practice with adolescents. Wiley series personality processes* (pp. 307-331). New York: John Wiley and Sons.

Tomlinson, R. and Peters, P. (1981). An alternative to placing children. Intensive and extensive therapy with "disengaged families." *Child Welfare* 60(2):95-103.

Tomm, K. (1984). One perspective on the Milan systemic approach Part II: Description of session format, interviewing style and intervention. *Journal of Marital and Family Therapy* 10:253-271.

Vargus, I.D. (1977). Supervision in social work. In D.J. Karpius (Ed.), *Supervision of applied training*. Westport, CT: Greenwood Press.

Voydanoff, P. (1990). Economic distress and family relation: A review of the eighties. *Journal of Marriage and the Family* 52:1099-1115.

Voydanoff, P. and Donnelly, B.W. (1989). Economic distress and mental health: The role of family coping resources and behaviors. *Lifestyles: Family and Economic Issues* 10(2):139-162.

Wang, M.C. and Gordon, E.W. (Eds.) (1994). *Educational resilience in inner-city America: Challenges and prospects.* Mahwah, NJ: Lawrence Erlbaum.

Waskell, C. (1996). Multidisciplinary teamwork in primary care: The role of the counsellor. *Counseling Psychology Quarterly* 9(3):243-260.

Watzlawick, P. Weakland, J., and Fisch, R. (1974). *Changes: Principles of problem formation and problem resolution.* New York: Norton.

Wells, S. (1981). A model of therapy with abusive and neglectful families. *Social Work* 26:113-118.

Whitaker, C.A. (1967). The graving edge. In J. Haley and L. Hoffman (Eds.), *Techniques of family therapy* (pp. 265-360). New York: Basic Books.

Whitaker, J.K., Kinney, J., Tracy, E.M., and Booth, C. (1990). *Reaching high-risk families: Intensive family preservation in human services.* New York: Aldine de Gruyter.

White, M. (1990). The externalizing of the problem. In M. White and D. Epston (Eds.), *Narrative means to therapeutic ends* (pp. 38-76). New York: Norton.

White, M. (1995). *Re-authoring lives: Interviews and essays.* Adelaide, Australia: Dulwich Center Publication.

White, M. and Epston, D. (1989). *Literate Means to Therapeutic Ends.* Adelaide, SA, Australia: Dulwich Centre Publications.

White, M. and Epston, D. (1990). *Narrative means to therapeutic ends.* New York: Norton.

Winnicott, D.W. (1971). *Playing and reality.* London: Tavistock Publications.

Wolin, S.J. and Wolin, S. (1993). *The resilient self: How survivors of troubled families rise above adversity.* New York: Villard Books.

Woodbury, M.A. and Woodbury M.M. (1969). Community psychiatrist intervention: A pilot project in the 13th Arrondissement, Paris. *American Journal of Psychiatry* 126:619-625.

Yamamoto, J. and Goin, M.K. (1966). Social class factors relevant for psychiatric treatment. *Journal of Nervous and Mental Disease* 142:332-339.

Zimmerman, J.L. and Dickerson, V.C. (1994). Using a narrative metaphor: Implications for theory and clinical practice. *Family Process* 33(3):233-245.

Index

Page numbers followed by the letter "f" indicate figures; those followed by the letter "t" indicate tables.